Coconut Oil For Health And Beauty

Cynthia Holzapfel
Laura Holzapfel

16
EasyRead Large

RHYW

Copyright Page from the Original Book

Cover design: Warren Jefferson
Interior design: Gwynelle Dismukes

Molecular illustrations in chapter 2 done with ChemSketch, version 5.0, Advanced Chemistry Development, Inc., Toronto Ont., Canada, www.acdlabs.com, 2003.

Inline molecules in figures 1-1, 1-2, 1-3, and 1-9 on pages 15, 16, and 23 from *Food Fats and Oils*, reprinted with permission from the Institute of Shortening and Edible Oils, Inc., 1750 New York Avenue, NW, Washington, D.C., 20006.

Published in the United States by
Book Publishing Company
P.O. Box 99, Summertown, TN 38483
1-888-260-8458 www.bookpubco.com

Printed in Canada
ISBN 1-57067-158-3
ISBN13 978-1-57067-158-6

12 11 10 9 8 7 6

Holzapfel, Cynthia, 1948-
Coconut oil for health and beauty / Cynthia Holzapfel, Laura Holzapfel.
p. cm.
Includes bibliographical references and index.
ISBN 1-57067-158-3
1. Coconut oil--Health aspects--Popular works. 2. Fatty acids in human nutrition. I. Holzapfel, Laura. II. Title.
QP752.F35H64 2003
613.2'84--dc22
2003020825

The Book Publishing Co. is a member of Green Press Initiative. We have elected to print this title on paper with 100% postconsumer recycled content and processed chlorine free, which saved the following natural resources:

23 trees	1,067 lbs of solid waste
8,313 gallons of water	2,003 lbs of greenhouse gases
16 million BTUs	

For more information visit: www.greenpressinitiative.org. Savings calculations thanks to the Environmental Defense Paper Calculator: www.papercalculator.org

TABLE OF CONTENTS

Introduction	ii
1: The Chemistry of Fats	1
2: The Role of Fats in the Body	16
3: Nutritive Benefits of Coconut Oil	32
4: The Antimicrobial Properties of Coconut Oil	49
5: Coconut Oil Beauty Tips	70
6: Coconut Facts & Tips	76
7: Recipes	93
Breakfast & Baked Goods	95
Soups & Salads	102
Main Dishes	105
Grains & Side Dishes	112
Desserts	119
Drinks	133
GLOSSARY	137
REFERENCES	142
Back Cover Material	152
Index	153

In appreciation

We would like to thank the following individuals for their suggestions, advice, and support:

Robert Gaffney, Omega Nutrition
Brian Silhavy, Tropical Traditions
Dr. B.I. Naddy
Brenda Davis, RD
William Shurtleff

and to Helen Housel,
mother and grandmother,
for her love of learning and sense of adventure.

Introduction

Why focus on fats?

The modern field of nutrition is a relative newcomer on the scientific scene. Although many ancient civilizations have maintained an awareness of how food contributes to health, it has only been during the last hundred years (and especially the last fifty years) that what we eat has become the subject of research science. Beginning with the discovery of the building blocks of life—the elements carbon, oxygen, and nitrogen—early scientists isolated minerals, such as calcium and iron, which also were noted as essential for good health. With the identification of vitamins in the early 1900s, scientific understanding of the role specific substances play in sickness and health increased exponentially.

Early on, scientists and health care practitioners were primarily concerned with nutritional deficiency, situations where people had difficulty getting enough calories or essential nutrients such as protein, vitamins, or minerals. Sometimes these deficiency problems were a result of poverty; other times they were related to a mineral deficiency in the soil or a lack of fresh produce. After World War II, the development of modern transportation systems and refrigeration increased the diversity of the food supply in developed nations so much that over-abundance became more of a problem than deficiency. Along with this increased abundance came an increase in chronic diseases, which eventually eclipsed infectious illness as the main cause of death. Deadly diseases, such as bacterial pneumonia and tuberculosis, had been greatly reduced by antibiotics; however heart disease (including coronary artery disease and high blood pressure), cancer, and diabetes increased in near epidemic proportions.

By some estimates, over 40 million Americans have some form of cardiovascular disease and more than 1. 5 million people die of heart attacks each year. Although recent reports on cancer mortality show that rates of death from cancer are on the decline, rates of cancers that are related to nutritional factors (specifically cancers of the breast, colon, prostate, and pancreas) have not declined as quickly as lung cancer, which is primarily caused by tobacco use. Furthermore, the current obesity epidemic is causing concern in all areas of health care. While the nutritional causes of these diseases are many and varied, studies have implicated the type and amount of fat in our diets as a top contender.

The conflicting information on diet and fats

Why does there seem to be so much conflicting information about the reasons some foods protect us from disease while others cause health problems?

Perhaps the most widely disseminated and confusing information concerns vegetable oils. In the '60s and '70s, polyunsaturated oils (such as corn oil) were widely touted as protective against heart disease, and people were frequently advised to switch from eating butter to margarine in order to lower cholesterol levels. Researchers now believe that diets high in polyunsaturated vegetable oils actually increase our chances of contracting heart disease, and the trans fats in margarine are implicated in a number of health problems in addition to heart disease. With all these contradictory guidelines, it's easy to see why some people have become cynical about any nutritional advice and have gone back to eating whatever suits their fancy.

Why would a particular food fall in and out of favor with nutritionists so quickly? It's important to realize that the tremendous growth in the number of nutritional discoveries that have been made in the last ten to fifteen years is unparalleled in almost every other field of science. The field of nutrition now involves many diverse scientific disciplines, such as genetics, immunology, molecular biology, pharmacology, and biochemistry. Nutritional science is like a newly discovered continent on which researchers are intrepid, modern-day explorers. These explorers are forced to reevaluate the information they gain about their discoveries as they press further into the inner reaches of this foreign shore.

Dean Ornish, MD, had celebrated success reducing heart disease in his patients using a diet consisting of low-fat plant foods (with the addition of some skim milk products). This success was duplicated by John McDougall, a physician practicing in Hawaii, and Caldwell Esselstyn, a cardiologist with the Cleveland Clinic, both of whom published influential studies showing that low-fat diets lowered cholesterol levels and improved the health of patients suffering from heart disease.

Other reseachers got much different results when studying high-fat diets. To some degree, studies of cultures whose eating habits have not changed much over the centuries provide us with some of the most reliable information on how different fats affect the development of chronic disease. When researchers moved beyond controlled studies and looked at how people ate in their own homes, they were surprised by the amount of fat was consumed. One of the most significant of these studies was Ancel Keyes' Seven Countries Study, which established a relationship between saturated fat, cholesterol, and heart disease. It's interesting to note that the lowest level of mortality from heart disease was found in Crete, where the level of fat consumption was actually quite high. Although the amount of saturated fat eaten on the island was low, so was the amount of trans fats. Studies done on the Polynesian islands of Pukapuka and Tokelau showed low levels of cholesterol and heart disease even though islanders ate significant quantities of saturated fat from coconut oil.

With any research conducted in the area of nutrition, the trick is trying to isolate which elements of the diet are most protective. Also, researchers still are not sure what role the genetic makeup of these populations (as well as any factors in their particular environment) may have in influencing how their diet affects their health. A number of experts have speculated that the practice of eating locally grown, whole foods may play an important part in maintaining a long, healthy life.

Why the interest in coconut oil?

For many years coconut oil was a common ingredient in baked goods and was used for frying. Because it is a stable saturated fat, it helped keep foods fresh. It didn't break down when used for fried foods.

However, when saturated fat was implicated as a possible cause for heart disease, all the saturated tropical oils, including coconut oil, palm kernel oil, and palm oil, earned the same unfavorable reputation as saturated animal fats. The Center for Science in the Public Interest, eager to expose areas of notable nutritional excess and deficiency, targeted the use of coconut oil in fried foods and movie theater popcorn. The result of this negative publicity was a sharp decrease in the use of coconut oil in commercial foods and consumer resistance to using it in their kitchens.

Proponents of coconut oil also cite how the American vegetable oil industry and other pertinent business interests were concerned about the commercial threat of coconut oil and may have exerted influence on public policy and scientific research to discredit it.

We believe coconut oil has many benefits, and we hope this book will clarify why we feel its revival is justified. We'll explain some of the chemistry of fats and oils to give you the background you'll need to understand how fats are used in the body for growth and health. Coconut oil is getting more attention from researchers because of its proven ability to reduce bacterial and viral infection, so we'll also review the results of some of this research. For those who want to learn more about how to use coconut and coconut oil, we cover everything from how to purchase fresh coconuts to where to buy quality coconut oil—plus we explain how to use coconut products in beauty formulas and include delicious recipes for every season and occasion.

Cynthia Holzapfel
Laura Holzapfel

1

The Chemistry of Fats

For some people, just knowing that the saturated fat from coconut oil has a different composition than saturates in meat and dairy products would be information enough. If your level of curiosity is satisfied by that statement and you're not sure you want to tackle the science of fat chemistry, don't feel you have to assimilate all the information in this chapter. You might prefer to skim the highlights, stop and learn a few terms, and go on to find out what health benefits you can gain from coconut oil.

However, if you're the curious type who needs to have all the facts, we hope you'll find this chapter informative. We've made our basic chemistry lesson very simple. It will enrich your understanding of how fats act in the body and how coconut oil works to provide nutritional benefits and protect against disease.

Some chemistry 101

There are well over one hundred elements that science has identified to date (an element is a substance made up of only one kind of atom). To understand how fats are formed, it's important to know how atoms bind together to form a molecule, the smallest piece of any substance that still maintains the properties of that substance. Early physicists compared the atom to a ping-pong ball with a small nucleus at the center and electrons circling around an outer shell. Today we know that the structure of the atom is much more complex than this simple model. It is composed of many small particles, some that have only recently been discovered, and others that have not yet been identified but whose influence can be detected. Also, electrons do not form a single shell-like layer around the nucleus but are grouped in several layers (the number of layers is relative to the number of electrons contained by the atom).

One method atoms employ to bind with other atoms is determined by the number of electrons those atoms hold in their outer layers. In order to be complete, an atom must have eight electrons in its outer layer. Only a few of the elements (the noble gases, such as helium, neon, and radon) already have all eight electrons in their outer layer. To complete this "rule of eight," most elements must share electrons with other elements. This sharing of electrons is called *bonding.* With some exceptions, when atoms share electrons, or form a bond, they each contribute at least one electron to this union; one atom does not simply give an electron to another atom. A bond that consists of two shared electrons, each belonging to a parent atom, is known as a *single bond.* In a *double bond,* each atom will contribute two electrons, for a total of four shared electrons.

The two principal elements involved in the chemistry of fats are carbon (noted by the symbol C) and hydrogen (H). The basic structure of any fat is a chain of carbon atoms. Carbon has four electrons in its outer shell and must share these electrons with other atoms to be complete. Therefore, carbon must share four bonds. In figure 1-1, each line represents a single bond with two shared electrons. (To make this easier to follow, think of an electron being at each end of the line between atoms.)

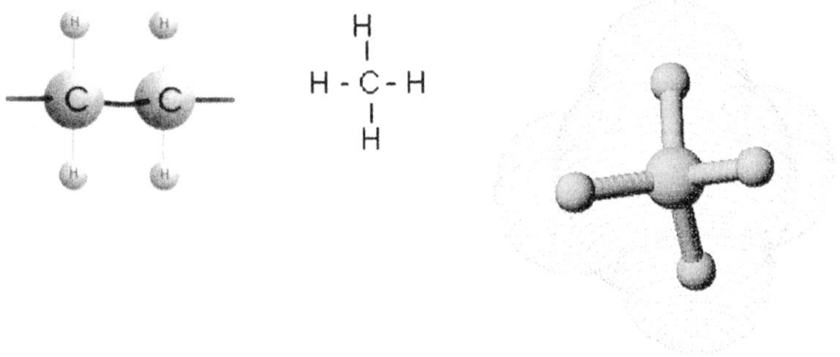

Figure 1-1: Examples of a single bond

In a double bond, each carbon will contribute two electrons with at least one other atom that also contributes two of its electrons (a total of four shared electrons). It's also possible for carbon to be linked by two double bonds to two other atoms. As a result of doubling up on the shared atoms, carbon would only have to share bonds with two or three other atoms, instead of the four atoms it must find if it only makes single bonds. Figures 1-2 and 1-3 show some examples.

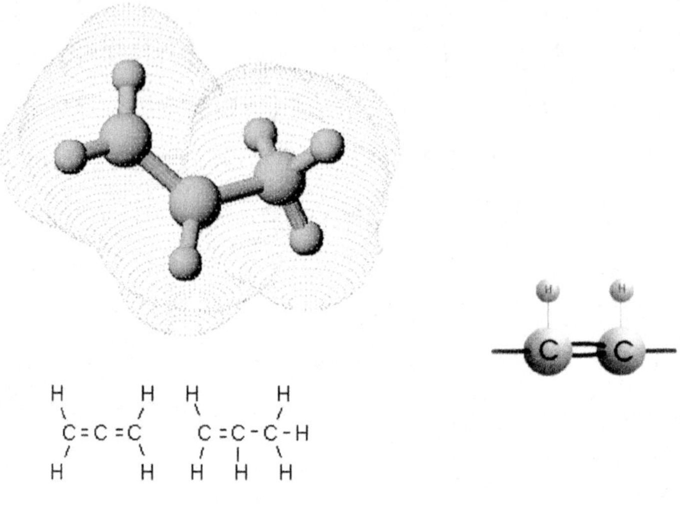

Figure 1-2: Examples of one double bond

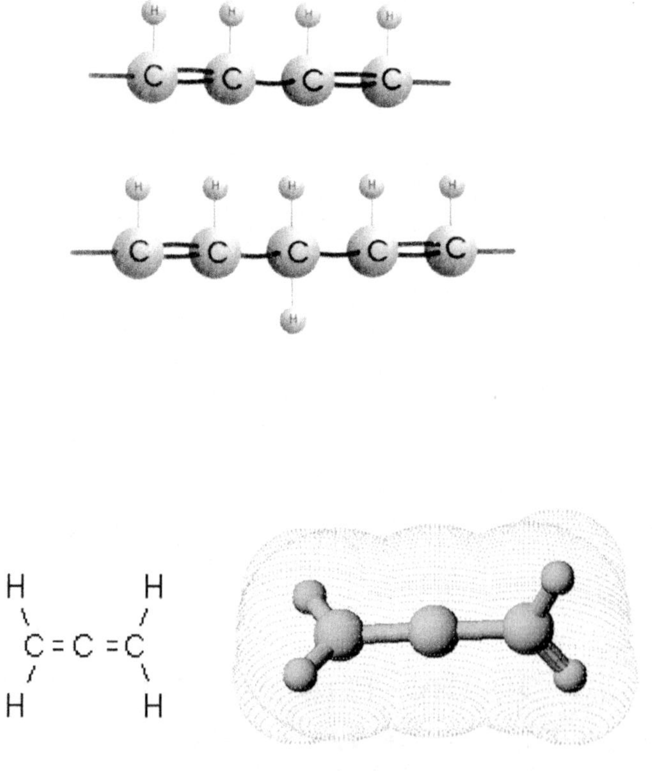

Figure 1-3: Examples of two separate double bonds

Carbon chains in fats

If a towel is soaked in water and cannot hold any more moisture, we say that is it "saturated." The same can be said about a row of carbon atoms that are not only linked to each other in a chain but are sharing the remainder of their necessary bonds with hydrogen atoms; the carbon chain is called *"saturated."* This is the origin of the term *saturated fat.* Figure 1-4 on the next page shows a saturated carbon chain.

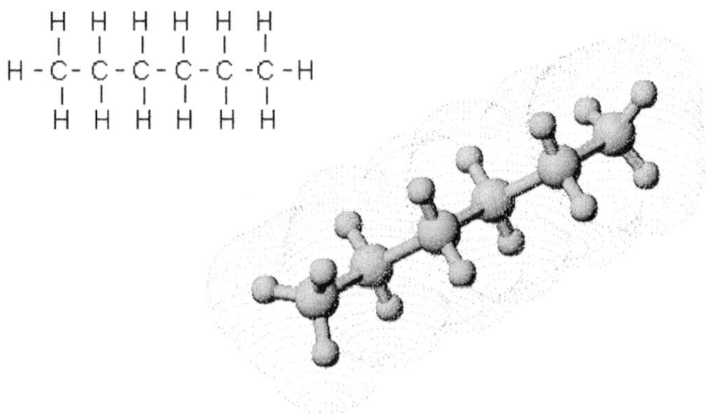

Figure 1-4: Saturated carbon chain

A carbon chain where at least two of the carbon atoms are sharing a double bond with each other in the chain instead of just one bond is called *unsaturated.* This is the basis of the term unsaturated fat. The simplest example of this is in a *monounsaturated fat,* where two of the carbon atoms share two bonds (four electrons) instead of one bond (two electrons). A monounsaturated fat would resemble a towel that is almost saturated but could hold a little more water before starting to drip. Figure 1-5 below shows an example of a monounsaturated carbon chain.

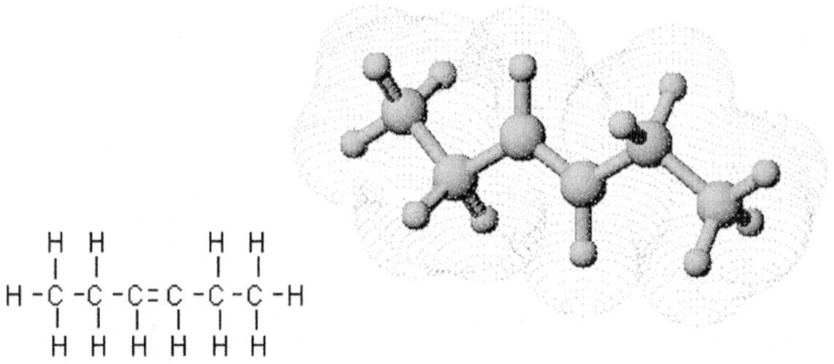

Figure 1-5: Monounsaturated carbon chain

A *polyunsaturated fat* has a chain of carbons where at least two of the carbon atoms are sharing two bonds with at least two other carbon atoms in the chain. This would result in a total of four or more carbons sharing double bonds. Figure 1-6 shows a polyunsaturated carbon chain:

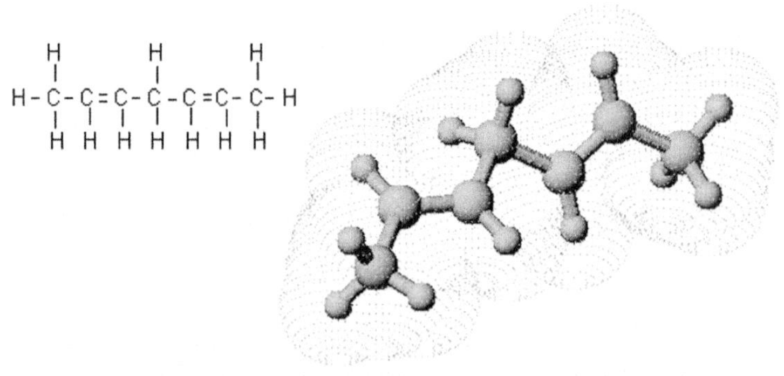

Figure 1-6; Example of a polyunsaturated carbon chain

In any sort of unsaturated fat (whether it is monounsaturated or polyunsaturated), a double bond creates a weak spot in the chain, making it more unstable. Although the carbon atoms are sharing enough electrons with other atoms to get their requisite eight electrons, a double bond between two atoms is not as strong as a single bond. At first glance it might seem that the more electrons two atoms share, the stronger those shared links would be, but the increased sharing of electrons leaves potential openings along the chain of atoms. A double bond creates a situation similar to a gap between two teeth or a window that's cracked open just a little. It increases the potential for more flow and the chance that another atom or interfering molecule might attract one of the shared electrons from the double bond.

A saturated fat is the most stable of the fats. It is less likely to lose, gain, or trade a bond along its carbon chain. One could say that carbon atoms are unhappy when they are only bonded to three other atoms. They would like to find a way to be singly bonded to four atoms.

From carbon chains to triglycerides

Both fats and oils are commonly referred to as *lipids.* The principal difference is that fats are solid at room temperature (like shortening), and oils are liquid at room temperature (like olive oil). Lipids are composed of the same basic groups: three fatty acids and one glycerol molecule. When fatty acids and glycerol combine, they are called a *triglyceride* (tri = three fatty acids, glyceride = glycerol). Fatty acids come in different lengths, and the length partially determines the properties of the specific lipid.

A fatty acid molecule is composed of a chain of carbons and hydrogens with an acid (carboxylic) group on the end, as shown in figure 1-7:

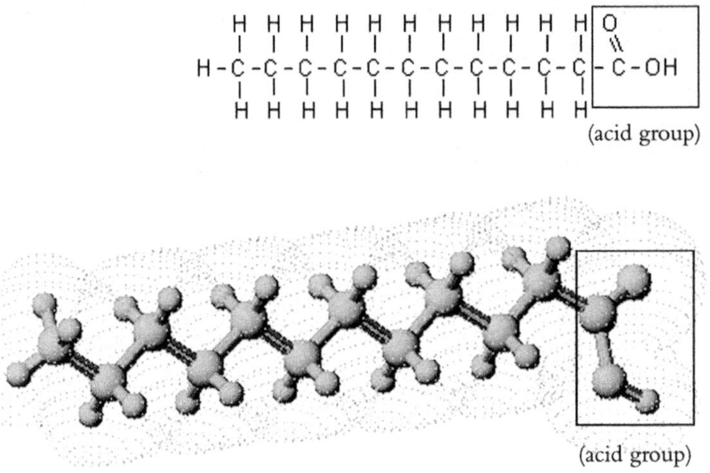

Figure 1-7: Example of a fatty acids molecule

How an acid group attaches to a carbon chain is quite complicated and can be done in a number of ways. For our purposes, it's enough to know that the acid group is formed when an oxygen atom and an oxygen-hydrogen molecule replace three of the hydrogen atoms at the end of a carbon chain, attaching to the carbon atom that remains.

The length of the chain and the number of double bonds (if there are any) and their position determine the type of fatty acid. For example, lauric acid, the principal fatty acid in coconut oil, has a twelve-carbon chain (this includes all the carbon atoms, even the carbon in the acid group). None of the bonds between the carbon atoms are double, so lauric acid is a saturated fat.

Here is a list of different fatty acids and the length of their carbon chains:

Fatty Acid	Number of Carbons	Common Food Source
Saturated		
Butyric	4	Butter
Caproic	6	Butter
Caprylic	8	Coconut oil
Capric	10	Coconut and palm kernel oils
Lauric	12	Coconut and palm kernel oils
Myristic	14	Nutmeg oil
Palmitic	16	Palm oil, other vegetable and animal fats
Stearic	18	Cocoa butter and animal fats
Arachidic	20	Peanut oil
Monounsaturated		
Palmitoleic	16	Animal fats
Oleic	18	Olive oil, other vegetable and animal fats
Erucic	22	Rapeseed oil (canola)
Polyunsaturated		
Linoleic (omega 6)	18 (2 double bonds)	Soy, corn, sunflower, and safflower oils

Fatty Acid	Number of Carbons	Common Food Source
Alpha-linolenic (omega 3)	18 (3 double bonds)	Flaxseed and hempseed oils
Gamma-linoleic (GLA)	18 (3 double bonds)	Black current seed and primrose oils
Arachidonic (AA)	20 (4 double bonds)	Animal fats
Eicosapen-taenoic (EPA)	20 (5 double bonds)	Fish oil
Docosahex-aenoic (DHA)	22 (6 double bonds)	Fish oil

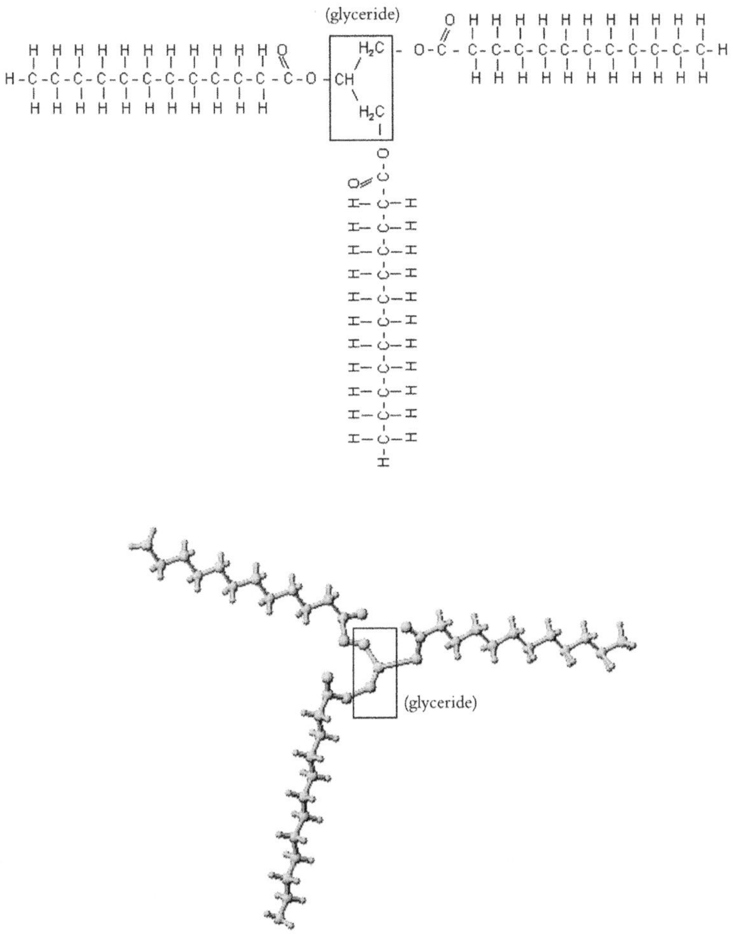

Figure 1-8: Example of a triglyceride made up of lauric acid, the principle fatty acid in coconut oil. Each fatty acid is attached to the glyceride. The hydrogen atoms have been removed from an end of each acid group, and the lone oxygen that is left has bonded to the glyceride.

Fatty acids with four or six carbons in their chain are known as *short-chain fatty acids.* Butter is a source for these fatty acids. *Mediumchain fatty acids* have eight to twelve carbons in their chains (although some researchers also include fourteen-chain fatty acids as medium-chain). Most of the fatty acids that make up coconut oil are medium-chain fatty acids. Fatty acids with fourteen or more carbons are called *long-chain fatty acids.* These make up the largest group of lipids—most animal fats and vegetable oils.

Chemically altered fats

TRANS FATS

For the most part, trans fatty acids are manufactured from polyunsaturated fats to have properties that more closely resemble saturated fats. Trans fatty acids were created in order to replace either saturated fats that were in short supply (such as butter during war times) or unstable polyunsaturated fats in baked goods (to prolong their freshness on supermarket shelves).

There are a few naturally occurring trans fats in some animal fats, but they are formed predominately by a process that requires heat and pressure to alter their chemical structure. As shown in figure 1-9 on the next page, a polyunsaturated fat has at least one double bond between two carbon atoms. The single hydrogen atoms that still are bonded to these carbons are on the same side of the carbon chain. The carbon chain bends at the point where the double bond occurs, angling in the direction of the two hydrogen atoms.

Because polyunsaturated fatty acids have this bended shape, they cannot pack together closely. Saturated fats, on the other hand, have no double bonds and no bend along their carbon chain. Because they are straight, they can pack together more densely. This characteristic explains why saturated fats tend to be solid at room temperature and unsaturated fats are liquid.

In the early 1900s, chemists were looking for a cheap alternative to solid fats. Modern oil processing techniques made liquid oils plentiful and inexpensive. Scientists discovered that liquid oils can be converted to a solid form if one of the hydrogen atoms attached to a double-bonded carbon is transferred to the opposite side of the carbon chain. As a result, the fatty acid straightens out, creating the desirable characteristics of a tightly packed saturated fat, even though it is fundamentally still an unsaturated fat.

There's a twist, however—both literally and figuratively. Although trans fats have the chemical composition of unsaturated fats, the altered position of the hydrogen atom creates a twist in the carbon chain, so that the atoms aren't aligned the same way they are in the unsaturated fat. This causes a problem when trans fats are utilized by the body. The sensitive systems that use fats for essential processes in the body recognize trans fats as unsaturated. But when they try to use trans fats the way they would use unsaturated fats, the altered chemical structure of the trans fats doesn't allow them to be used properly. They take up the space normally reserved for unaltered unsaturated fats and block certain processes from occurring. We'll talk more in the next chapter about the health implications trans fatty acids.

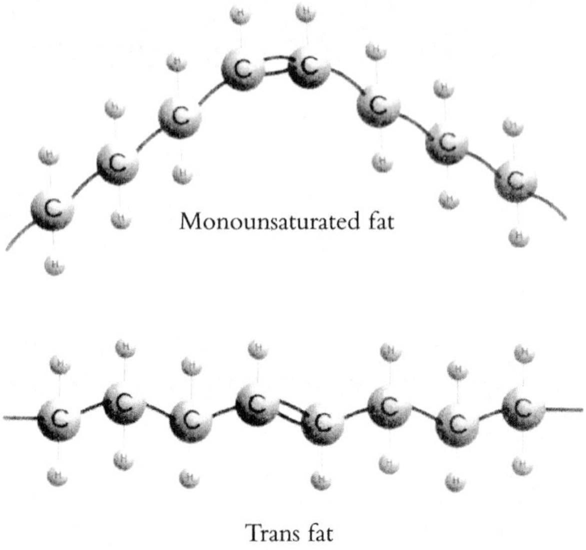

Figure: 1-9

HYDROGENATION

Hydrogenation is another artificial process used to transform liquid oils into solid fats. During this process, heat, pressure, and hydrogen gas are used to add hydrogen atoms to the double bonds of unsaturated carbon chains, creating a straightened chain without any unstable bonds. Partial hydrogenation occurs when only some of the double bonds are filled with hydrogen atoms. By filling only some of the gaps along the carbon chain, chemists can control the solidity of the finished product.

The process of hydrogenation disrupts the original chemical composition of unsaturated fats. A number of the chains are broken down instead of being filled with hydrogen, resulting in altered substances that are harmful to the body. It's impossible to completely control the chemical reactions that occur during hydrogenation or ensure that only a minimal amount of these unwanted molecules is produced. Trans fats also are created during hydrogenation.

The case for avoiding chemically altered fats

We've grown accustomed to the way our foods are manufactured using chemically altered trans fats and hydrogenated fats. Food processors love them, as it makes their products less prone to spoilage, and manufacturers can more closely control how these foods look and taste. In some cases these altered fats are much less expensive than the solid fats they replace. But this financial savings comes at great cost to our health. Let's take a look at how fats are used in the body to understand why.

2

The Role of Fats in the Body

Fats are our principal source of energy. They contain about nine calories per gram, whereas carbohydrates and protein contain four calories per gram. Simply put, protein builds our tissues, and carbohydrates provide us with an immediate source of energy that's not only useful in terms of physical exertion but is essential for brain function. Accumulated fats in the body provide a storage repository of energy in times of famine. It may be difficult to imagine the need for such a survival mechanism in modern times of plenty, as many of us struggle with our desire for high-calorie treats. However, the ability to store fat was absolutely essential for our ancestors, whose food supplies were not always dependable or nutritious. It is so important for the body to have a supply of fat to draw on (for all the reasons that are discussed later in this chapter), that even during times of extreme weight loss, the body tries to retain a certain amount of fat.

Because fats are digested more slowly than protein or carbohydrates and are such a concentrated source of calories, they help diminish feelings of hunger, letting us know when we've eaten enough. The body's "appestat," or appetite thermometer, is regulated to keep us from constantly overeating. Although diets high in refined carbohydrates make it easier for us to override this regulator, in the ancient diets of our ancestors, the consumption of a certain amount of fats triggered a signal that meant "enough calories for now, thank you."

An adequate layer of fat under our skin also protects us from the cold. Often we become more interested in high-fat foods as the shorter days of autumn prompt our bodies to prepare for winter, making that time of year more difficult for dieting. The practice of midwinter holiday partying definitely is related to this natural drive to store more fat! Surrounding vital organs and cushioning bones, fat also provides protection from the jostling of daily activities and the shock of impact when walking, sitting, and handling hard objects.

Fats also shape who we are, because they play a role in forming secondary sex characteristics. Men tend to put on more abdominal fat than women, and women have larger deposits of subcutaneous fat (the fat that lies directly beneath the skin) and fat in the buttocks, thighs, and breasts. It's often thought that the particular distribution of fat in a woman's body is related to her biological role in childbearing, ensuring that she'll have an adequate supply of fat in her breast milk and plenty of calories for growing a baby.

Essential fat for bodily processes

In order to understand how fats function in the body, we need to know how they interact with other compounds. Fats can travel throughout the body by themselves in the form of triglycerides—the molecule containing three fatty acids that was described in the previous chapter—or in combination with other substances to perform certain functions. First, we'll provide a general overview of some of these combinations. Then we'll explore what their role is in the body.

Fats can combine with carbohydrates to form *glycolipids.* Glycolipids are an integral part of cell membranes. They are, in a sense, nature's gatekeepers, recognizing what substances should be allowed into a cell. They also form part of the structure of the nervous system, forming receptors that handle electrical signals sent throughout the body (signaling pathways). People who are afflicted with Tay-Sachs disease, a fatal disease of the nervous system, have inherited the inability to make an enzyme needed to metabolize certain glycolipids.

When fats combine with phosphate, they form *phospholipids.* Lecithin is one example of a phospholipid. These molecules transport fats in and out of cells and help to keep fats moving in the bloodstream. Like glycolipids, phospholipids also are important components of cell membranes. They form the "skin" of cell membranes, providing structure and helping to keep membrane proteins in place.

When fats combine with protein, they form *lipoproteins.* Lipoproteins are capable of carrying fat and cholesterol in and out of the bloodstream, because they have a water-soluble outer surface that allows them to flow easily in fluids and a fat-soluble core that combines well with fats.

Fatty acids synthesize hormones called *prostaglandins,* which affect everything from inflammation, blood pressure, blood clotting, and other functions of the circulatory system. Certain hormones made from omega-6 fatty acids increase these conditions; those made from omega-3 fatty acids reduce them. (The omega fatty acids cannot be formed by the body from other fats, so they are known as *essential fatty acids.*) A good balance between these two types of fats helps regulate body functions and ensure good health.

Finally, fats metabolize vitamins A, D, E, and K and the carotenoids (such as beta-carotene, which can be formed into vitamin A). Vitamin A plays an essential role in maintaining the outer layers of tissues, both within the body and in the skin, and ensures the growth of healthy bones. Vitamin D is also a bone builder, helping to absorb and metabolize calcium and phosphorus. Vitamin E is an antioxidant, protecting tissues from free radical damage and tumor development. Vitamin K helps with blood clotting and bone formation. Carotenoids also are antioxidants and help protect the immune system. Fats help the body absorb these vitamins, transporting them through cell membranes. The body also uses cholesterol to synthesize vitamin D.

How are fats metabolized in the body?

The digestion of fats is not a neat process where fats simply are broken down into smaller and smaller substances that ultimately are absorbed by cells. Components of fats are broken apart and then reformed all along the metabolic process from the stomach to the liver. At various points along the way, different cells draw off fat molecules for use. Sometimes triglycerides are broken down into free fatty acids (fatty acids that are not attached to glycerol or any other molecule), only to have those fatty acids later recombined as triglycerides for use in other areas of the body. Ultimately, most fats are absorbed six to eight hours after they are eaten.

Although the digestive process begins when we chew our food, the first significant digestion of fats occurs in the stomach, where fats are separated from other nutrients in foods by various enzymes and broken up by another enzyme, gastric lipase.

Most digestion of fats happens in the upper small intestine, where they are emulsified by bile salts produced by the gallbladder so the fats will combine with water and can be transported into the blood stream. Intestinal and pancreatic enzymes, called lipases, break down triglycerides into *monoglycerides* (glycerol + a fatty acid), which are then split further to produce free fatty acids and glycerol.

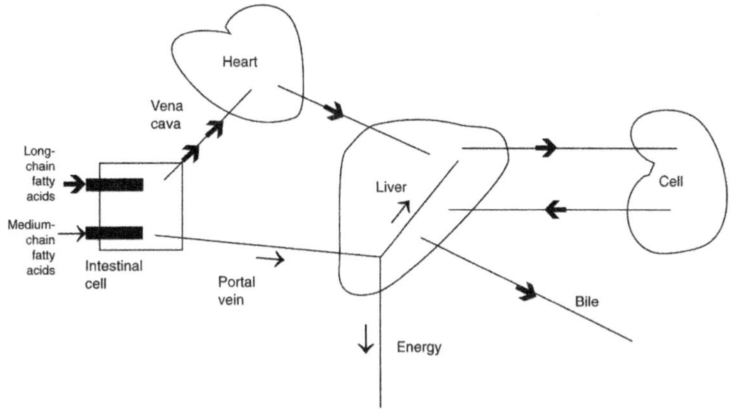

Figure 2-1: The metabolism of medium-chain and long-chain fatty acids, showing the different pathways taken through the liver and into cells.

Short- and medium-chain fatty acids (those with twelve carbons or less) can be absorbed directly into the bloodstream and transported to the liver by the protein in blood (albumin). More complex fats and fatty acids will not dissolve in water as easily and must recombine with some of the water-soluble substances mentioned in the previous section: proteins (to become lipoproteins), carbohydrate (as with glycolipids), or phosphorus (phospholipids). These substances can then move into the bloodstream and proceed to the liver.

Most fats are metabolized in the liver. From there, new triglycerides, as well as phospholipids and cholesterol, are carried through the bloodstream by either high-density lipoproteins or low-density lipoproteins. You may be more familiar with these terms from their abbreviations: HDL and LDL. The density refers to the amount of protein in these molecules, as protein has a greater density than does fat. LDL transports cholesterol to artery walls to repair damage; HDL removes cholesterol from artery walls and returns it to the liver so it can be eliminated from the body if not needed.

HDL = high-density lipoprotein = more protein than lipids

LDL = low-density lipoprotein = more lipids than protein

You'll often see HDL and LDL referred to as "cholesterol," but this is shorthand somewhat for "cholesterol carried by high-density or low-density lipoproteins."

Fats that are not metabolized shortly after digestion are stored in fat cells under the skin (adipose tissue), as is any excess carbohydrate. A certain amount of carbohydrate can be stored in muscle cells and in the liver for quick use, but once the liver has taken in all it can hold, it converts this carbohydrate into stored fat.

Are all fats metabolized and used the same way?

In our discussion on how fats are metabolized, we saw that not all fats take the same route through the digestive or metabolic process. Short- and medium-chain fatty acids, those with twelve carbons or less, are absorbed directly into the blood and transported to the liver on albumin (blood protein). Most, but not all, of these short- and medium-chain fatty acids are saturated fats, from both animal and plant sources. They are used quickly and primarily as a source of energy, as opposed to longer saturated and unsaturated fatty acids. Because of this, people with liver problems find shorter chain saturated fatty acids easier to digest, as they require less work by the liver to break up and recombine for use in the body.

Long-chain fatty acids (fatty acids with fourteen carbons or more) are converted into triglycerides in the intestine and take more work to transform into a structure that can be absorbed in the bloodstream. Most, but not all, of these long-chain fatty acids are unsaturated fats. Some of the triglycerides they form have special functions in various cells; most of them go to the liver where they are broken down into fatty acids once again for use in the cells. These fatty acids have a special role helping to keep the cell membranes more fluid. Because they are more unstable than saturated fats, these molecules will attract oxygen atoms, creating an environment that is inhospitable to bacteria and viruses and playing a role in the movement of electrical impulses in the body.

The longer the carbon chains in the saturated fat, the greater the tendency these fat molecules have to aggregate or cluster and hold together. Their positive role in the body is to help form the structure of cell membranes. On the down side, they also form plaques, the sticky substances that gather around injured areas in artery walls and contribute to clogged arteries.

What about trans fats?

Since the early 1900s, the use of trans fats has been on the rise, both in processed foods and in the home. As explained in chapter one, trans fats are natural fats that have been artificially modified to make them more stable and solid. At the time they were developed they were seen as an inexpensive alternative to solid animal shortening. After World War II, most of the hydrogenated oils were used in margarines. With the growing commercialization and processing of the American food supply, hydrogenated fats played an important role in keeping foods fresher on supermarket shelves and allowing for the development of inexpensive fast foods. Even though coconut oil could have filled much of this niche without having to be processed, the presence of a large supply of vegetable oils in the U.S. encouraged the growth of artificially solid vegetable fats.

Although the body tries to use trans fats in the same way it would use the unmodified fat from which the trans fat is made, trans fats are too chemically different from natural fats to fill the same role. Fortunately, some parts of the body, especially the brain (and the placenta of unborn babies) and certain enzymes, can recognize a few of the differences between trans fats and natural fats and are capable of rejecting the trans fats.

Because trans fats have a more rigid structure than the natural oils from which they are made, they interfere with normal cell processes. Instead of properly fitting into the fluid structure of cell membranes, more solid trans fats disrupt the natural nutrient flow in and out of the membranes and allow substances into and out of cells that are detrimental to cell health. Unlike natural fats, trans fats cannot provide the same biochemical reactions that contribute to the flow of electrons necessary for the release of energy and the proper functioning of the nervous system. This disruption can cause problems with maintaining a regular heartbeat, proper firing of neurons, cell division, functioning of the senses, mental stability, and sustaining overall well being.

Trans fats interfere with the enzymes that play a role in metabolizing the essential fatty acids, omega-3s and omega-6s, into more complex fats. These fats are important to large organs and hormone function. This interference also limits the production of prostaglandins, the complex essential fatty acids that control the balance and regulation of blood pressure and blood stickiness.

The body also tries to convert as many of the trans fat molecules into energy as it can. But it cannot perform this conversion as quickly on trans fats as it can with natural fats, so the rate of metabolism of fatty acids will be reduced. Also, if trans fats comprise a sizeable portion of fats in the diet, the body tries to use them for the essential functions that are normally handled by natural fats, instead of whatever natural fats are available.

The role of cholesterol

Although cholesterol is not a fat, it's so often mentioned along with discussions of fat that many people think they are one and the same. Cholesterol actually is a waxy substance created in our bodies from small molecules of acetate that result primarily from the breakdown of fats and sugars, and in some circumstances, protein. We also can get cholesterol from eating animal products; it is never found in plant foods.

Cholesterol has gotten a bad reputation over the years because of its association with heart disease. But like many natural substances, cholesterol is not all bad. There is evidence that some people (such as the elderly) cannot make all the cholesterol they need and may benefit from the addition of some cholesterol in their diet.

Healthy individuals produce the cholesterol they need for their bodies to function. Cholesterol is essential for helping cell membranes retain their structural consistency. The fluidity of these membranes is constantly changing relative to the types of fatty acids present in the body. Unsaturated fatty acids tend to make cell membranes softer and more fluid; saturated fats make the membranes more rigid. Cholesterol flows in and out of cell membranes, creating just the right balance to keep the membranes at the correct consistency during changing conditions. This balance is so important that each cell has the capacity to create its own cholesterol. Similar to its role in keeping cell membranes strong, cholesterol also plays a role in healing damaged tissue. It's used by the body, along with calcium and collagen, to form scar tissue.

Cholesterol is also a building block for vitamin D and certain hormones, especially the hormones that regulate sexual functioning: estrogen, progesterone, and testosterone. Cholesterol is used to make stress hormones, as well. When the body is under stress, more cholesterol is created to form adrenal hormones, a primal physical response that helps prepare us to either fight or flee the source of stress.

Is cholesterol the cause of heart disease?

There definitely is evidence that high levels of cholesterol in the blood are associated with the hardened arteries and arterial blockages that lead to heart disease, but there is disagreement among experts as to whether eating foods high in cholesterol causes this condition. It would seem to make sense that a person could lower the amount of serum cholesterol (cholesterol in the blood) by consuming less cholesterol in the foods they eat. But in study after study, it's been difficult to show a significant correspondence between cholesterol consumption and serum cholesterol levels.

Some researchers have focused on trans fats as a cause of high cholesterol levels, theorizing that the presence of these fats crowds out natural fats that would help the body maintain normal, healthful amounts of cholesterol. Other experts are looking at whether an overabundance of free radicals (unstable molecules that are created during normal biological processes) can create artery damage that then is repaired by cholesterol. An accumulation of cholesterol at any one site of damage could cause blockage in that blood vessel. The lack of certain vitamins and other antioxidants may lead to higher levels of free radicals and in turn create conditions that would lead to the production of more serum cholesterol.

Looking beyond cholesterol as a cause of heart disease, some experts have pointed to high levels of omega-6 fats (found in cottonseed, corn, safflower, soybean, and sunflower oils) as a trigger for increased blood pressure, inflammation, and blood clots. The use of oils high in omega-6 fats has been promoted widely over the last thirty years as a healthful alternative to saturated fats, but recently the wisdom of this recommendation is coming under fire from some sources.

Do saturated fats raise cholesterol levels?

Saturated fats have been implicated for many years as a cause of increased cholesterol levels. When measurements of serum cholesterol (cholesterol levels in the blood) were first done, they only read the total of both good HDL and bad LDL and assumed the presence of both indicated high levels of cholesterol. Now that testing has become more sophisticated, researchers look more at the balance of these two types of lipoproteins and note whether a substance raises cholesterol only when levels of HDL are increased or whether LDL levels also are higher. In some cases, certain foods lower total cholesterol levels, but only by lowering good HDL quite a bit while simultaneously raising levels of bad LDL.

For a long time saturated fat also was thought to increase the incidence of heart disease, but the data collected from several significant studies on saturates and coronary disease do not confirm a direct correlation. Subsequently, some cardiovascular researchers are questioning this long-held belief. Prominent in this group of researchers is Walter Willett, MD, DrPH, of Harvard University, himself a longtime proponent of the relationship between saturated fat and heart disease. Willet participated in a study of over 43,000 health professionals who had no prior incidence of heart disease or diabetes, where a conclusion was:

> "Diets high in saturated fat and cholesterol are associated with an increased risk of coronary disease, but these adverse effects are at least in part explained by their low fibre content and association with other risk factors. Benefits of reducing intakes of saturated fat and cholesterol are likely to be modest unless accompanied by an increased consumption of foods rich in fibre."[1]

Although saturated fats, especially the saturated fats in animal products, tend to clump together or "aggregate" in the arteries, eating saturated fats may not in and of itself put us at risk for blocked arteries, heart disease, and stroke. Certainly eating high levels of particular vegetable oils high in omega-6 fatty acids also can put us at risk for conditions that often lead

---

1 Ascherio, Alberto, et al. "Dietary fat and risk of coronary heart disease in men," BMJ (1996): 313:84-90.

to heart disease (high blood pressure, inflammation, blood clotting) and even cancer (cell proliferation). Eating a diet that is high in essential omega-3 fatty acids from whole food sources such as flaxseed, hempseed, walnuts, and even greens, provides a good balance for diets that include saturated fats and other polyunsaturated vegetable oils.

In the end, heart disease may result from any number of causes, and what produces heart disease in one individual may not affect another individual. A recent study at the Cleveland Clinic that examined 120,000 heart patients concluded that smoking, diabetes, high blood pressure, and high cholesterol are the most important overall risk factors for heart disease. The best we can say at this point is that eating a diet high in natural, unprocessed foods and not participating in behaviors that are risky to our health are the best defenses against arterial damage.

3

Nutritive Benefits of Coconut Oil

Coconut oil has many good qualities in its favor. As a solid, saturated fat that doesn't easily become rancid at room temperature or break down with high heat, it can be used to enhance baked goods and cook or fry foods. Besides being a valuable ingredient in food preparation, coconut oil has specific health benefits that make it worthwhile adding to our diets.

Topping the list is the fact that coconut oil makes an excellent replacement for trans fats in processed foods. Hydrogenated vegetable oils that are solid at room temperature form the basis of margarine and vegetable shortening and can be found in hundreds of bakery items and other foods where a solid fat delivers the richness and mouth-feel that people enjoy and have come to expect. At the time, nutritionists championed the replacement of solid animal fats (which they believed were a major contributor to coronary artery disease) with what they then thought were more healthful, artificially solid vegetable fats.

Over the years, however, trans fats became implicated in a growing array of health problems, primarily heart disease—the very ailment for which they were thought to be protective. A number of studies showed that trans fats increased bad cholesterol (LDL) and decreased good cholesterol (HDL). In a double-blind study published in 1992, researchers in the Netherlands looked at the effects of replacing animal fats and hydrogenated oils with palm oil, another saturated tropical oil similar to coconut oil.[1] (In a double-blind study such as this, participants are divided into two groups, each group consuming a different diet. Halfway through the study the two groups switch diets so that it's easier to determine whether the test results are a result of the diets or other factors particular to the participants themselves.) Although the diet using palm oil didn't lower total cholesterol levels, it did lower LDL cholesterol by 8 percent and increased HDL cholesterol by 11 percent.

A 2001 study done in the Netherlands showed that replacing foods containing trans fats with those containing saturated fats (particularly foods in which lauric acid, the primary fat in coconut oil, made up about one-third of the saturates) also improved HDL cholesterol levels.[2] The use of lauric acid gave even better results than in the studies where palmitic acid (the primary fat in palm oil) was the main saturated fat. Although palm kernel oil (which is different from palm oil) was the high-lauric saturated fat used in this study, the researchers commented that coconut oil is also a rich source of this fatty acid, suggesting that they would get similar results with coconut oil.

Inflammation, digestion, and other health problems

Coconut oil may be helpful in reducing inflammation, the body's response to infection. A British study tested the response of mice to a five-week diet that was either low in fat or high in one of the following oils: olive, safflower, coconut, or fish oil. The mice on all the diets were exposed to pathogens and their physical responses were studied. The results showed that both fish oil and coconut oil did more to diminish inflammation in the mice than any of the other fats they were fed, leading the researchers to believe that "both these fatty acids might be useful therapies in acute and chronic inflammatory diseases."[3]

Ideally, we might be able to improve the overall quality of the nation's diet if we were able to alter food preferences and reduce the use of foods requiring any solid fats. However, changing these preferences would probably be very difficult. On a positive note, these studies from the Netherlands indicate that there is much that could be gained if fat sources such as coconut oil were used instead of trans fats and other saturated fats. The work of Finnish researchers indicates that diets high in polyunsaturated fats (especially the omega-6 fatty acids and trans fats found in margarine) might contribute to the increased incidence of allergies in children.[4] It is thought that polyunsaturated fats might increase inflammation and lead the immune system to trigger allergic reactions. Although asthma in particular, and immune responses in general, probably are caused by a complex series of factors of which diet is only a part, the growing amount of information on how dietary fat is associated with allergies makes it an important aspect to consider.

Because medium-chain fatty acids are more quickly digested than long-chain saturated fats, they are often a good choice for individuals who have digestive disorders or more delicate digestive systems (such as infants or seniors). Mother's milk has a high content of lauric acid, leading nutritionists to consider coconut oil a good food for babies due to its high proportion of lauric acid. A number of studies have been conducted on the healthful properties of adding coconut oil to infant formula. In one such study done at the University of Iowa in 1996, researchers compared how well fat and calcium were absorbed by infants.[5] The infant formulas they used contained either palm oil (which is comprised predominantly of palmitic and oleic acids, both unsaturated fats) or coconut oil. They found a significant improvement in absorption when the babies were fed formula rich in coconut oil.

Coconut oil also may be beneficial for people who suffer from Crohn's disease, a disorder marked by inflammation of the intestines, as well as those with ulcerative colitis, a similar disease affecting the colon. Research has been done showing that the anti-inflammatory properties of coconut oil are effective at reducing the irritation created by Crohn's disease. In addition, coconut oil's antimicrobial properties (which are explored more in the next chapter) may be effective in fighting the bacteria and viruses often cited as a cause of Crohn's disease, stomach ulcers, and other ulcerative diseases of the intestinal tract. Coconut oil is readibly assimilated by people who struggle with digestive diseases, making it easier for them to eat nutritious foods and regain their health.[6]

Another potential use for coconut oil may be the treatment of benign (noncancerous) enlarged prostate in men. Currently a popular and successful herbal treatment for this condition is the use of saw palmetto berries. These berries contain a substance that inhibits DHT, which is derived from testosterone and increases in men as they age. DHT is thought to be responsible for cell growth in the prostate, leading to its enlargement. It is believed that the active ingredient in saw palmetto berries is a lipid extract containing medium-chain fatty acids. Therefore, it is possible that coconut oil, with its high content of medium-chain fatty acids, may also have a positive effect on prostatitis and enlarged prostate.[7]

Higher metabolism and weight loss

Most of us have accepted that when it comes to the calorie content of fat, all fats are created equal: nine calories per gram. Surprisingly this is not the case.

Coconut oil actually contains slightly fewer calories (about 10 percent less) than other fats. Does this mean that switching to a diet where all our fat comes from coconut oil will help us shed pounds quickly? Probably not, as a 10 percent reduction in calories just from our fat sources won't add up to much:

1,800-calorie diet with 30 percent calories from fat
= 540 calories from fat.
Less 10 percent calories from fat
= a reduction of 54 calories per day.

These fifty-four calories per day are roughly equivalent to what we'd expend by walking briskly for seven or eight minutes while swinging our arms vigorously to maintain our pace or riding a bike at a leisurely speed for ten to fifteen minutes. Undeniably, this amount of exercise would be great for our heart and circulatory system, and we'd feel the benefits from the exposure to fresh air and sunshine. But we would need to sustain this activity for a much longer period than a few minutes to see significant weight loss. Although a reduction in the consumption of fifty calories a day would contribute to a slow, steady weight loss, to try to accomplish this by eating only coconut oil as a fat source would eliminate other important fats in our diet, especially essential fatty acids.

Coconut oil may contribute to weight loss in ways other than reduced calories. An excellent report by Marie-Pierre St-Onge and Peter Jones of McGill University, Quebec, Canada, on whether medium-chain fatty acids could be used to prevent obesity was published in 2002 in the *Journal of Nutrition*.[8] The authors presented an overview of almost thirty studies on the various effects of medium-chain fatty acids on metabolism, satiety (the sensation of fullness after eating), body fat, and body weight.

In their compilation, most (but not all) studies showed an increase in metabolism with diets high in medium-chain fatty acids where 30 to 40 percent of calories came from fat. One study showed an increase initially, but it was not sustained for more than a few weeks.

When it came to weight loss, men seemed to have the advantage—for reasons not clear to the researchers. When fed diets high in medium-chain fatty acids, the metabolism of the men rose sufficiently to achieve an average weight loss of about 16 kilograms (thirty-five pounds) a year. For the women, this loss was closer to five and one-half kilograms (twelve pounds) a year. Because these studies were small and brief, there still is much more work to be done to prove conclusively that medium-chain fatty acids could effectively increase metabolism to sustain long-term weight loss. However, there is promise, and hopefully a renewed interest in coconut oil will spur more researchers to conduct larger and more lengthy studies.

In terms of satiety (how well a meal makes us feel full or satisfied), the effects of medium-chain fatty acids were somewhat less clear but still indicated they may play a role in decreasing appetite. Subjects who ate more medium-chain fatty acids for breakfast tended to eat less for lunch. There was little correlation between the type of fat eaten for breakfast and how much subjects ate for dinner, leading to speculation that the best results might be obtained if medium-chain fatty acids were eaten throughout the day.

There also is a possibility that coconut oil can contribute to decreased stores of white fatty tissue, the layer of fat below the skin that so often accumulates around the waistline (as opposed to the brown, fatty adipose tissue that surrounds internal organs). In a 1998 study conducted in Spain, researchers varied the fat and calorie content in diets fed to rats, enriching one of the test diets with coconut oil. Their results showed that the diet high in coconut oil stimulated a cell component called UCP1 (uncoupling protein), essential for the processing of food into energy in cells. In this way coconut oil actually helped to reduce subcutaneous fat stores in the rats in this study.[9]

Is it risky to eat saturated coconut oil?

It's safe to say that few people had any opinions about the healthfulness of coconut oil until a negative assessment of it by the Center for Science in the Public Interest (CSPI) was widely publicized in the early 1990s. The focus of this publicity was the use of coconut oil on movie theater popcorn, as well as its addition to baked goods. CSPI has conducted many informative campaigns exposing nutritional deficiencies in the processed foods available in supermarkets and the high calorie content of restaurant dishes. However, this is one instance where the watchdog organization may have jumped on the anti-saturated fat bandwagon before doing its homework. At the very least, a consideration of the health of large groups of people who have made coconut oil their principal fat source for generations would lead to a very different conclusion about whether coconut oil should be demonized.

Proponents of coconut oil point out that many of the studies condemning the saturated fat in tropical oils have been done using refined tropical oils. This would eliminate some of the healthful properties found in the unrefined oil traditionally consumed by native populations in tropical areas. There also were a number of animal experiments conducted where coconut oil was blamed for increasing cholesterol levels and heart disease. But in these experiments the animals also were on diets that restricted the amount of essential fatty acids needed to help prevent the incidence of these health problems, so the results of the studies probably were more reflective of a lack of essential fats than a problem with coconut oil.[10]

A number of more positive studies have been carried out in India and Southeast Asia, where consumption of coconut oil is at some of the highest levels in the world. In southern India, fresh and dried coconut and coconut oil are staples in the diet. The traditional diet in India is much lower in fat than Western diets, yet coronary artery disease is significantly on the rise, much in the same way that it is in regions of the world where diets are high in fat, especially saturated fat. P.D. Kumar, a researcher from the South Indian state of Kerala, compared a group of people with coronary artery disease with a control group of healthy individuals and discovered that the consumption of coconut oil in both groups was about the same.[11] The presence of coconut oil in the diet did not increase the risk for arteriosclerosis; in fact, when the amount of coconut meat, or kernel, in the diet was increased, harmful LDL cholesterol levels actually dropped.

In Malaysia, researchers looked at the effects of controlled diets containing proportionally high amounts of palm oil, corn oil, or coconut oil.[12] They found that while coconut oil raised the total amount of cholesterol in the blood, it did so by raising the ratio of good HDL cholesterol to bad LDL cholesterol. Although both palm oil and corn oil reduced total cholesterol, they also reduced the proportion of HDL cholesterol—a factor that researchers feel is a more important risk factor for heart disease. Similar results were seen when the fatty acids found in coconut oil—lauric acid and myristic acid—were increased in the diets of healthy men. Again, although the total levels of cholesterol increased slightly, it was due in large part to the increase of healthful HDL cholesterol, a positive factor for health.[13]

Agronomist P.K. Thampan has written extensively about the research studies that evaluate coconut oil consumption and health in Southeast Asia. He noted that in Sri Lanka alone, the average consumption of coconuts is about ninety each year per person (about one-quarter of one coconut every day)—and that's just for whole coconut. The amount increases to 120 coconuts each year per person when the amount of coconut oil consumed is taken into account, making Sri Lanka an excellent place to study coconut oil's effects. Thampan describes a study of sixteen young men who were fed a diet where coconut oil and other coconut products were the main sources of fat. Then the same men were fed a diet where the principal fats were from dairy products and corn oil. Measurements of the blood lipid levels of the study's participants showed that the corn oil diet lowered total cholesterol levels but also lowered levels of good HDL cholesterol. However, the diet high in coconut fat not only kept total cholesterol at a healthful level (around 180), it kept HDL levels high relative to LDL levels.[14][15]

Perhaps the most quoted study on this subject was carried out by Ian Prior on the Polynesian islands of Pukapuka and Tokelau, where coconut oil is a major source of fat in the diet. It contributes 35 to 56 percent of calories (compared to U.S. recommendations of 30 percent of calories from all fat sources).[16] Because of this, the amount of saturated fat in the diet is quite high, but the incidence of cardiovascular disease is very low. Cholesterol levels ranged from 170 to 180 on Pukapuka to between 210 and 215 on Tokelau (where overall fat consumption was the greatest). Most importantly, heart disease was not a common health problem for the people on these islands, even with the large amount of saturated plant fat they consumed.

The case against polyunsaturates

Eating a diet too high in polyunsaturates may be more harmful to health than eating the saturated fats in coconut oil. Several recent studies show that extracting certain oils from their source and consuming those oils without the protective nutrients that accompanying them in their natural state may be unhealthful for several reasons. Nuts and seeds contain flavonoids and phenolic acids that fight cancer and heart disease. The fiber in nuts and seeds also helps reduce the incidence of diabetes (as long as the total fat intake is moderate). Perhaps most importantly, the protective shells and skins on nuts and seeds minimize how quickly the oils inside degrade or spoil. Once polyunsaturated oils are isolated from their whole foods source, they tend to break down and become unstable. The result of this instability is the formation of free radicals, the harmful substances that were described in chapter two. These unstable molecules scavenge throughout the body for stable molecules they can raid to get the oxygen atoms they need for stability. The result is cell damage in the body.

In nature, polyunsaturated oils come packaged with healthful antioxidants that help prevent the degradation of these oils and the formation of free radicals. Common antioxidants in plant foods with a high oil content are vitamin E, flavonoids, and phenolic acids. Studies in India have shown that when there is an increase in the consumption of polyunsaturated oils high in omega-6 fatty acids and levels of antioxidants in the diet are low, there is an increase in certain ailments, especially hardening of the arteries and diabetes.[17] However, if the amount of omega-3 fatty acids in the diet (found in fish, flaxseeds, hempseeds, and certain tree nuts) is high relative to the amount of omega-6 oils (in a ratio of 1 to 4, or even 1 to 2), the incidence of these diseases is much lower.[18] When coconut oil is substituted for oils high in omega-6 fatty acids, it has a beneficial impact on the ratio of omega-6s to omega-3s and helps improve health in a variety of ways. These include better insulin utilization in people with diabetes and a reduction of high blood pressure, the presence of protein in the urine (kidney dysfunction often associated with diabetes and high blood pressure), LDL levels, and possibly gallstones and cancerous tumors. So not only is it important to concentrate on getting a higher level of omega-3 fatty acids in the diet, but omega-6s can be reduced when stable oils such as coconut oil are used to replace unstable polyunsaturated oils, resulting in a more favorable balance of omega fatty acids.

Coconut oil as a part of a healthful, high-fiber, plant-based diet

Much of the research on the relationship of saturated fats and heart disease points to the possibility that saturated fats and cholesterol in animal products may play more of a role in causing health problems than saturated fats in plant foods. However, as researchers uncover more information on the role of nutrition in health, it often becomes less clear why various foods cause or prevent disease. Heredity plays a key role in shaping our biology and to what degree each of us is susceptible to certain health problems. Although the consumption of cholesterol and saturated animal fat can lead to high cholesterol levels and heart disease, there are scores of people whose cholesterol levels are not adversely affected this way.

Many medical professionals believe that the simple theories about whether saturated fats and cholesterol are bad for health depend on whether these substances are eaten as whole foods (or as part of a diet rich in whole foods) or if one's diet is largely made up of refined foods. Even the 1996 Harvard University study that was quoted at the end of chapter two indicated that eating whole plant foods might play a significant role in protecting individuals from heart disease, whether or not they eat foods high in cholesterol or saturated fat.

For many years the focus of nutritional recommendations for people with diabetes was to reduce the amount of sugar and other carbohydrates they consumed. In more recent years, diabetes research has become more sophisticated, and there is growing concern about the amount of fat contributing to increased incidence of diabetes. With the growing epidemic of obesity, it is impossible to ignore the fact that being overweight increases our chances of contracting diabetes, affirming that no singular food group is the culprit when it comes to the development of this terrible disease. An interesting discovery researchers have made as they measure the effects of a variety of foods on blood sugar levels is that unprocessed, high-fiber foods do the best job of regulating blood sugar, regardless of whether these foods are primarily carbohydrates, fats, or protein. This revelation also makes a good case for embracing a wide variety of whole plant foods in the diet, rather than focusing on one food group or nutritional component as being a destroyer or proponent of good health.

Does the inclusion of fresh coconut in the diet help boost the healthful properties of coconut oil? P.K. Thampan makes a good case for considering that the benefits of coconut oil can be optimized by including it in a whole foods, plant-based diet when he states:

> All the edible components of coconut contribute substantially to the dietary calories of people in the major coconut growing and consuming countries. The edible components are also good sources of protein, fibre, and minerals. This could be the reason why people consuming large amounts of coconut and coconut oil in a varied diet in different parts of the world do not demonstrate hypercholesterolaemia[high cholesterol levels] and coronary heart disease.
>
> The only limitation in the dietary use of coconut oil is its low content of essential fatty acids. This deficiency will not, however, become manifest when people consume a normal diet containing cereals, pulses [beans and other legumes], roots and tubers, fish etc. which are good sources of these acids. Coconut oil and coconut kernel [coconut meat] as dietary components sustain optimum levels of vitamin E in people besides causing enhanced secretion of insulin and utilisation of blood glucose.[19]

We support this conclusion that using coconut oil—or any good-quality oil—is enhanced when it's a part of a whole foods, plant-based diet. We hope that the recipes in section entitled "Recipes" will help you discover new ways to incorporate coconut oil and other coconut products into a variety of dishes your whole family will enjoy. At the same time, these delicious dishes will help you enhance the nutritive benefits of coconut oil.

COMPOSITION OF COCONUT OIL

acid	%	carbon chain length
lauric	50	12
myristic	18	14
caprylic	8	8
palmitic	8	16
capric	7	10
oleic	6	18 (monounsaturated)
stearic	2	18 (saturated)
linoleic	2	18 (diunsaturated)

4

The Antimicrobial Properties of Coconut Oil

In the past 150 years, there have been significant advancements in the fight against infectious diseases. Even with this progress, outbreaks still persist and previously unknown diseases continue to surface. One such instance occurred in 1993 in Milwaukee, Wisconsin, with the contamination of the municipal water supply. It resulted in an outbreak of cryptosporidiosis, a parasitic infection in the intestine that affected an estimated 400,000 people. Roughly 4,400 of those who were infected required hospitalization.[1]

Although scientists had predicted that the fight against infectious diseases would have been won by now, the arrival of new viruses and the reemergence of previously defeated illnesses continue to plague the medical community. In the 1992 Institute of Medicine report, *Emerging Infections: Microbial Threats to Health in the United States,* it was noted that the death rate for infectious diseases rose 58 percent from 1980 to 1992.[2] Besides the ability of microbes to adapt and change, the reasons listed for this increase included the escalation of international travel for people, animals, and other traded goods, changing land use patterns, human demographics, and the breakdown of public health infrastructures to deal with infectious disease problems.

The problem of antibiotic resistance

A major factor in the increase of hospitalization and death rates from infectious diseases is the rise in antibiotic resistance in different types of bacteria. Many people expect to get an antibiotic each time they visit the doctor, as if it was the magic bullet for any ailment. Unfortunately, bacteria and other microscopic organisms can adapt so effectively that they can resist the drugs that are used to fight them. As a result, doctors have had to resort to using stronger and stronger antibiotics in order to cure infectious diseases.

How do bacteria overcome such potent medicines? If you have a bacterial infection, your doctor may start you on an antibiotic. If you take this antibiotic incorrectly (by not taking all of it or delaying doses too frequently), it may kill many, but not all, of the bacteria in your system. The few bacteria that remain could be ones that become resistant to the antibiotic you were using because they were able to survive the partial doses of antibiotics you took.

These bacteria will start multiplying and soon you'll feel sick again. Unfortunately, the antibiotic you had taken will be useless against this new infection. Once a bacterium has resisted an antibiotic and survived, it will be able to reproduce. It does this by splitting itself and forming two sister cells that are identical to the original bacterium cell (with the exception of any random mutation that might occur). These sister cells will pass on to all of their offspring the ability to resist the antibiotic you took. The replicas will continue to divide, creating offspring that are exactly like the parent bacterium. The generation time—the time it takes a bacterium to divide—can be a matter of minutes (with bacteria such as E. coli) or up to a few days. Most bacteria have a generation time of about two hours, so the potential for new infections can increase quickly.

Once you've become a host to a more potent and rapidly growing strain of bacteria, your doctor will have to put you on an antibiotic that can destroy these hardier microorganisms. Unfortunately, this has some drawbacks. The stronger the antibiotic you take, the greater the chance that the helpful bacteria in your intestinal system also will be destroyed. Even though antibiotics wipe out harmful invaders, they are foreign substances in the body as well, and their presence places extra stress on the liver and other cleansing organs.

There also are unpleasant side effects associated with antibiotics. Some of these effects are common to a number of medications; other problems are unique to specific drugs. The most frequent side effects of several common antibiotics are allergic reactions, which can sometimes be life threatening, nonallergic rashes, severe skin rashes, diarrhea, vomiting, and abdominal cramping. Any time we take an antibiotic we increase the risk that harmful bacteria will become resistant to that particular medication. If we increase the potency of the antibiotics we take, we also increase the risk of harboring more potent bacteria.

Bacteria are more complex than most of us realize. Some bacteria have the ability to share information with other organisms, including how to become resistant to different antibiotics. (This sharing process-would be similar to what would happen if bacteria were able to mate!) Theoretically, this ability would allow the bacteria that causes an earache to share information with the bacteria that causes the stomach flu. Therefore, the problem of antibiotic overuse is made more complex, as the chance for resistance isn't limited to the strain of microorganisms we are attempting to overcome, but to any number of other strains in our system, as well.

The relevance of this becomes more apparent in the context of how much illness is caused by infection. The Centers for Disease Control and Prevention (CDC) estimates that food-related pathogens alone generate around 76 million known cases of illness per year in the United States, resulting in 325,000 hospitalizations and more than 5,000 deaths. Of these, approximately 62 million infections and 3,200 deaths are caused by unknown organisms. In a recent report on food-related illness and death, the CDC stated that "more than two hundred known diseases are transmitted through food."[3] Even if the harmful bacteria we consume don't cause us to become ill at the time, chances are increasing that they are resistant to antibiotics and could pass on this resistance to a different and extremely dangerous organism. For example, we might be harboring a relatively benign form of E. coli virus, but if that virus comes in contact with a resistant organism, it could assimilate the information it needs to become a virulent form of E. coli, capable of causing a life-threatening illness that does not respond to antibiotics.

Antibiotic resistance has become endemic. In 1995 the American Medical Association studied this sweeping trend and concluded that "The global increase in resistance to antimicrobial drugs, including the emergence of bacterial strains that are resistant to all available antibacterial agents, has created a public health problem of potentially crisis proportions." The reemergence of tuberculosis (TB) illustrates the dangers of antibiotic resistance. In order to cure an infection of tuberculosis, the patient must take antibiotics for six to nine months, a therapy regime that often is not followed correctly. This has created an opportunity for tuberculosis to become a serious modern health problem—more significant and treacherous than it has been in the last seventy years. The global occurrence of TB is increasing at the rate of about four percent every year.

Antibiotic use in the meat industry

There also is considerable overuse of antibiotics in animal feed. For the past fifty years, farmers have fed cattle, pigs, and poultry low levels of antibiotics with the hope that this would reduce the infections caused by their cramped living quarters. In 1998, the European Union instituted recommendations proposed by the World Health Organization (WHO) and banned the use of antibiotics as growth promoters in the food animal industry. (These same antibiotics are commonly prescribed for the treatment of human infections.) In the WHO's *Report on Infectious Diseases 2000,* it was noted that introductory research done in Germany and Denmark corroborated that the ban of avoparcin as a growth enhancer in chickens has lessened the occurrence of vancomycin-resistant enterococci, not only in the birds themselves, but also in the human population as a whole.

Workers in the meat-packing industry regularly come in contact with resistant microbes as a result of handling animal carcasses in slaughterhouses and often develop illnesses that only can be cured with very strong antibiotics. When they become ill, packing plant workers have an increased chance of spreading these resistant germs to their family and friends. Meat-packing plants traditionally have had a poor record for maintaining safe, sanitary conditions, both for their workers and during the processing of the product itself. Meat easily is contaminated in these less-than-ideal conditions. All it takes is one viable bacterium to start a whole colony, so it's easy to understand why the combination of lax standards and antibiotic resistance is extremely dangerous.

Controlling viruses

Eighty percent of illnesses caused by known pathogens are initiated by viruses. Vaccines have contributed immensely to the eradication of many viruses. But to be effective a vaccine must be administered before we get sick, and only a select number of viruses even have associated vaccines. Although there are antiviral drugs on the market, not one of them effectively destroys the viruses in order to cure the illnesses they cause. All antiviral drugs do is slow the growth of the viral invasion; our bodies still must use their natural defenses to fight off the infection.

Our intention is not to cause undue concern with this information. At one time or another, nearly all of us have been afflicted with bacterial or viral illnesses that were not life-threatening. If our immune systems were working properly, we were able to fight off these illnesses with little, if any, use of antibiotics. But the growing overuse of antibiotics, and the subsequent rise of antibiotic resistance, should encourage all of us to investigate other ways to protect ourselves from microbial contamination and illness.

The healing properties of coconut oil

Coconut oil may help prevent illness or decrease its adverse effects once it strikes. In countries where coconut oil has been used for generations, it's considered an effective remedy for healing wounds. Some coconut industry experts are working to have coconut oil officially classified as a *nutraceutical,* a dietary supplement or food that protects against or treats chronic diseases while contributing beneficial nutrients.

Coconut oil actually can boost the functioning of our immune systems, unlike unsaturated oils high in omega-6 fatty acids that can weaken our immune systems by increasing inflammation and promoting cell proliferation. Coconut oil has even been shown to protect from six dangerous mutacarcinogens (cancer-causing agents that interfere with DNA), including benzpryine (found in cigarette smoke and diesel exhaust), azaserine, and nitrosamines (found in cigarettes and possibly in cooked meats cured with sodium nitrate). In the sections that follow, we'll explain how lauric acid and myristic acid, the primary medium-chain fatty acids in coconut oil, have been found to be protective against disease-causing microbes, including bacteria, viruses, funguses, yeasts, and protozoa. It's true that coconuts themselves are susceptible to bacteria and funguses. But once we ingest coconut oil, the triglycerides that are formed from this oil can become germ-killing molecules through the process of digestion that we describe in section entitled "How are fats metabolized in the body?". Mediumchain fatty acids are effective against many pathogenic organisms. Many microbes that are resistant to drugs that are used to fight infection may be overcome by the fatty acids in coconut oil. Eating foods with coconut oil may even prevent us from becoming infected by foodborne pathogens.

MICROORGANISMS THAT ARE DESTROYED BY MEDIUM-CHAIN FATTY ACIDS

Lipid coated bacteria	Lipid coated viruses
Chlamydia trachomatis	Cytomegalovirus
Dental plaque	Epstein-Barr
Gram-positive organisms	Hepatitis
Group A streptococci	Herpes simplex
Group B streptococci	Herpes viridae
Group F streptococci	Human immunodeficiency virus (HIV)
Group G streptococci	Human Herpes Virus-6A
Helicobacter pylori	Human lymphotrophic virus-1
Hemophilus influenzae	Influenza
Listeria monocytogens	Leukemia
Neisseria gonorrhoeae	Pneumonovirus
Staphylococcus aureus	Rubeola
Staphylococcus epidermidis	Sarcoma
Streptococcus agalactiae	Syncutial
Streptococcus mutans	Vesicular stomatitis virus
	Visna virus

How coconut oil works against microbes

Eighty percent of the medium-chain fatty acids in coconut oil have antimicrobial properties. Lauric acid, capric acid, caprylic acid, and myristic acid can interfere with the functioning of many harmful microorganisms. Of all of these, lauric acid, the main component of coconut oil, has shown the greatest capability to defend against viruses and most bacteria.

Many bacteria and viruses are embodied in a capsule made up of lipids. This lipid coating protects microorganisms from drying up when they are outside of our bodies. The coating also can help an invading organism infect us, much like a burr would stick to a furry surface. By adhering to our skin, mucous membranes, and internal organs, the bacterium or virus can evade our bodies' immune defenses as if it had a bullet-proof vest. Once inside our bodies, bacteria and viruses use lipids similar in structure to the medium-chain fatty acids in coconut oil to maintain this protective capsule coating. If our diets includes coconut oil, we'll have an increased chance that invading organisms will draw on these medium-chain fatty acids for their lipid coatings rather than from other fats. Unfortunately for the bacteria and viruses (but fortunately for us), medium-chain fatty acids do not maintain the integrity of this coating as well as other lipids do. This causes the lipid membrane that protects invading organisms to disintegrate around them. The increased permeability of this membrane allows the entrance of molecules that bacteria and viruses would rather keep out; it also allows the release of molecules they would rather keep in. The result is a situation similar to the breakdown of our own skin.

If we have a high concentration of medium-chain fatty acids in our bodies, we will have an extra line of defense protecting us from invading organisms. Our skin is continuously enriched by sebaceous glands that release protective oils. These oils prevent our skin from drying out and becoming more susceptible to infection. The composition of this oil reflects the lipids we consume: the more medium-chain fatty acids in our diets, the more medium-chain fatty acids we'll have on our skin. A higher concentration of lauric acid on our skin can even help fight off the bacteria that cause pimples and acne.

As we mentioned previously (see section entitled "From carbon chains to triglycerides"), the lipids in coconut oil are made up of triglycerides, or three fatty acids connected to a glyceride molecule. When we eat any fat, the triglycerides it contains are broken down. Some of the fatty acids break free from the triglyceride completely to form a lone free fatty acid. In other instances, a single fatty acid strand may remain connected to the glyceride molecule to form a monoglyceride (one fatty acid with one glyceride). The monoglycerides that are formed from the medium-chain fatty acids in coconut oil are the most potent at destroying bacteria and viruses. Out of all the free fatty acids, lauric acid is the most potent against many bacteria and viruses, though all medium-chain fatty acids show some ability to destroy these organisms. Palm kernel oil also contains lauric acid, and some companies have even gone so far as to synthesize a dietary supplement form of lauric acid. But coconut oil is still the most plentiful and inexpensive source of readily available lauric acid.

Coconut oil can be a great tool for defeating infectious bacteria. It has been shown to defend against the bacteria that cause staph infections, toxic shock syndrome, ulcers, several sexually transmitted diseases, meningitis, and stomach upset, and it reduces dental carries up to 80 percent. Though medium-chain fatty acids primarily affect gram-positive bacteria, they also are effective against strains of gram-negative bacteria. (Gram-positive bacteria have a simpler common cell wall composition and structure than gram-negative bacteria.) Worldwide, there are approximately fifty million new cases every year of *Chlamydia trachomatis* (the most common sexually transmitted bacterial disease); this includes around four million cases in the United States alone. A study done in Iceland on the effectiveness of medium-chain fatty acids against *Chlamydia* found that though high concentrations of capric acid were slightly more effective at reducing the numbers of all viable bacteria, lauric acid was much more effective specifically against

Chlamydia when both lauric and capric acids were used at a lower concentration.[4] The concentration of lauric acid used in this study more closely approximates the level we would obtain through the consumption of coconut oil.

Coconut oil and ulcers

Stress was once thought to be the main cause of ulcers. Although stress can be responsible for the onset of many illnesses, it now has been shown that the bacterium *Helicobacter pylori (H. pylori)* is the principal cause of chronic gastritis and about 90 percent of peptic ulcers. Treatments with antibiotics have shown promise, but unfortunately the percentage of infections that return is very great (mostly due to people not taking the medications correctly). The side effects of the treatment are unpleasant, leading many people to misuse the drugs given to them. As a result, doctors are seeing more and more antibiotic resistance from *H. pylori* bacteria.

The greatest advantage to fighting organisms with medium-chain fatty acids is that bacteria and viruses don’t commonly develop a resistance to them, regardless of the levels of medium-chain fatty acids in our bodies. The reasons for this are not yet clear to researchers, but one theory is that the medium-chain fatty acid’s effect on the very structure of invading organisms is too great for the organisms’ adaptive abilities to overcome.

Research has revealed another interesting key relating the success of coconut oil to the fact that it is saturated. When a monounsaturated form of lauric acid was tested along side the saturated form, it was shown that the bactericidal activity (how well it destroyed bacteria) of the saturated form was several thousand times more effective than its monounsaturated counterpart.[5] Also, although the monoglycerides of several medium-chain fatty acids were effective against bacteria, lauric acid was the only free fatty acid shown to be effective at destroying *H. pylori.* When the triglycerides of any fat are broken down, two free fatty acids, but only one monoglyceride, can be formed. So even though monoglycerides may be useful for fighting infection, the abundant presence of free fatty acids (such as lauric acid) may be the most important factor in determining which substance is most effective.

Lauric acid will still work against *H. pylori* even in the acidic conditions found in the stomach. Although stomach acid is strong enough to kill off many unwanted organisms, it isn't effective enough to destroy all infectious bacteria and viruses. In laboratory conditions, studies were done with acid solutions containing *H. pylori* showing that the addition of monocaprin and lauric acid effectively destroyed much of these bacteria. In fact, an acidic environment actually increased the potency of these free fatty acids against *H. pylori.* Because of this, we might expect a similar result in the acid conditions of the stomach.

Coconut oil and yeast infections

Not only could coconut oil reduce our dependence on antibiotics; it also may help maintain a healthful balance of intestinal flora. One of the discouraging side effects of drug treatment is that helpful bacteria are destroyed along with harmful bacteria. Certain "friendly" bacteria actually are needed to maintain health; for instance, they aid with digestion and produce an acidic waste substance that reduces yeast levels in the body.

Candida albicans is a type of yeast that normally lives in small numbers around the oral cavity, lower gastrointestinal tract, and female genital tract. When the body's defenses are lowered, an overgrowth of yeast can cause many problems and discomforts, including those listed on the next page.

The body's immune system works in concert with bacterial organisms that compete with the yeast for living space. Many infections caused by *Candida* occur when a dose of broad-spectrum antibiotics kills off helpful bacteria. Coconut oil may not only reduce the need for antibiotics, but the fatty acids in coconut oil also help destroy *Candida albicans* cells themselves.

Conditions that may develop from a yeast infection

abdominal pain
acne

adrenal problems
arthritis
bad breath
burning tongue
canker sores
colitis
congestion
constipation
cough (nagging)
depression
diarrhea
fatigue
headaches heartburn (persistant)
hyperactivity
hypothyroidism
impotence
itching (dermal and rectal)
kidney and bladder infections
memory loss
mood swings
muscle and joint pain
night sweats
numbness in the face or extremities
PMS
prostatitis
sinus congestion
sore throat
tingling sensations
vaginitis
white spots on the tongue and in the mouth

The same team of researchers who investigated the effect of capric and lauric acid on *Chlamydia* also studied how free fatty acids and monglycerides affected three different strains of *C. albicans.* They found that capric acid and lauric acid were the only two free fatty acids tested that had any substantial effect.[6] As it was against *Chlamydia,* capric acid was the most effective when free fatty acids were at a high concentration. However, lauric acid was the most efficient when the concentration of free fatty acids was lowered. When oleic acid (found in olive oil) and palmitoleic acid (found in butter fat) were tested, there was no significant difference in the reduction of viable yeast cells between those two free fatty acids and the untouched control.

Can coconut oil help in the fight against HIV and AIDS?

HIV and the associated disease AIDS affect countless people around the world, whether rich or poor, young or old. The choice of treatment, whether it's a drug cocktail or a more holistic approach, is a very personal and sometimes passionate decision for anyone who is afflicted with these illnesses. Reducing the amount of HIV in the body has been a promising way to abate the onset of AIDS.

An HIV-infected individual may live many healthy years before the disease progresses. Since the pandemic appearance of HIV, much money and time have been poured into research for drugs and other treatments to fight it. The unique qualities of HIV have made this fight more difficult. The way HIV replicates causes it to mutate more than most viruses. The many variations of the virus may not all be susceptible to the same drugs, which increases the possibility of resistance to the drugs used against them. Researchers in the Netherlands have assessed more than 1,600 blood samples of HIV positive people (28 percent female, 72 percent male) in seventeen European countries over the past four years. They found that as many as 10 percent of the recently diagnosed cases may include HIV forms that are resistant to some drug treatments.[7] In order to overcome these complications, a drug cocktail is often the treatment of choice. The use of these drug combinations has been credited for the decline in AIDS deaths in many wealthy nations.

Unfortunately, most of these drugs have undesirable side effects, including appetite reduction, nausea, muscle wasting, and displaced fat deposits that can lead to high cholesterol levels. Sadly, this increase in cholesterol can cause fatal heart attacks and lead to premature death before AIDS complications set in years later. These side effects have led numerous patients to seek out alternative treatments.

For many individuals, there are few treatment options. The United Nations Program on HIV and AIDS accurately projected that by January 2000, 34 million people would be living with HIV or AIDS—95 percent of these individuals would be in developing nations and 75 percent would be in Africa. Unfortunately drug cocktails are not readily available in less developed countries, and when they are, they are very expensive, easily reaching costs of over $15,000 per person each year. These areas of the world would greatly benefit from an inexpensive treatment alternative.

Coconut oil not only has the potential to be an effective tool for fighting HIV, but it also may help ease the symptoms of AIDS and the troublesome side effects of the drugs used to treat this illness. In addition, both coconuts and coconut oil are more readily available than many medications and much less expensive. HIV might be destroyed by coconut oil in much the same way as coconut oil destroys other susceptible bacteria and viruses.

Recently there has been much discussion and research on how the human herpes virus-6A (HHV-6A) can work synergistically with HIV to promote the onset of AIDS. It does this mainly by decreasing the amount of a specific lymphocyte (CD4) and destroying lymph nodes. A study by Knox and Carrigan in Wisconsin found that "The A variant of HHV-6 was found to be the predominant form of the virus present in the lymph node biopsies from all of [the tested] HIV-infected patients."[8] Fortunately, HHV-6A is one of the viruses killed by the medium-chain fatty acids found in coconut oil. HIV and HHV-6A incorporate medium-chain fatty acids into their protective lipid coating, which then disintegrates around them. One study concluded that, "The anecdotal reports that coconut oil does have an anti-viral effect and can beneficially reduce the viral load of HIV patients. The positive anti-viral action was seen not only with the monoglyceride of lauric acid but with coconut oil itself ... With such products, the outlook for more efficacious and cheaper anti-HIV therapy is improved."[9] In the same study, eleven out of fifteen subjects gained weight, ranging from four and one-half to fifty pounds.

The recommended amount of coconut oil in a therapeutic dose is three and one-half tablespoons per day. This equals the amount of oil found in approximately one-half of one coconut (about one cup grated), or forty-five milliliters (twenty-two grams) of monolaurin. Monolaurin capsules can be helpful, but the same amount of monolaurin can be obtained by eating coconut oil, which contains other beneficial medium-chain fatty acids.

Coconut oil may deactivate many of the inauspicious infections known to be a common complication for people who are HIV positive. It also may help the body maintain a healthful weight, a significant consideration for patients with HIV, AIDS, and other diseases that can cause wasting. Coconut oil could help undernourished individuals gain weight, while not adding excess to someone with a weight problem. During an initial study of the effect of coconut oil and monolaurin on HIV positive patients, three out of a group of fifteen developed AIDS (a CD4 count less than 200) in the first three months of therapy. One died of an AIDS complication two weeks after the study began, but one had fully recovered by the sixth month and the other was quickly recovering normal CD4 and CD8 counts. The two that recovered also had gained weight on this therapy.[10]

Coconut oil also can provide nutritional support during treatment. It is easily digested, high in calories (as are all oils), and known for providing energy more readily than other high-fat sources. Coconut oil has a very light flavor and a creamy texture, so it is convenient to incorporate in recipes such as soups, smoothies, baked goods, oatmeal cereal, and many other foods. It also may help improve overall immune system health and provide an extra defense against other opportunistic organisms.

Looking toward the future

A startling 2003 Harvard study showed that antibiotic use may be on the decline for the first time, especially for childhood illnesses. This offers some hope that we may be able to win the battle against antibiotic resistance. With the growing interest in alternative treatments for both chronic and acute illnesses, there certainly may be a place for coconut and coconut oil to be used with success. The nutritional stigma against coconut oil seems to be under scrutiny, and with it more research into its nutraceutical potential may follow.

5

Coconut Oil Beauty Tips

It's no accident that people living in regions where coconut oil is used both in the diet and for body care have beautiful skin and hair. The healthful properties of coconut oil are not only apparent internally but help promote a radiant glow all over.

Protecting yourself from free radical damage, both externally and internally, will help you avoid lines and wrinkles and extend your potential life expectancy. As we explained in chapters two and three, free radicals are unstable molecules that cause unwanted chemical reactions in the body. They can damage proteins, fats, cell membranes, and vital DNA, and contribute to the acceleration of the aging process.

Because of their chemical structure, unsaturated oils are more prone to free radical damage. In their natural state as part of whole nuts, seeds, and grains, they come packaged with protective antioxidants that limit free radical damage. When unsaturated oils are removed from their plant sources, they become more susceptible to a chemical chain reaction that degrades their quality. Because it is a stable saturated fat, coconut oil is not broken down by free radicals. When you use it to replace unsaturated fats in your foods or apply it to your skin, you reduce the opportunity for free radical damage and enjoy its anti-aging benefits.

The antimicrobal properties of coconut oil also extend to the skin and help you look more healthy and beautiful. As we mentioned in chapter four, coconut oil has been shown to help combat acne and promote healing.

Skin care

We experience dry skin more often after being out in the sun or during the winter months when the air inside and outside our homes is much lower in humidity than other times of the year. Dry skin also can be more of a problem as we age. Even people who have had very oily skin for much of their lives can experience dry skin on their legs and arms (where there are fewer oil glands than other areas of the body) in their later years.

Coconut oil can be a wonderful, natural alternative to expensive (and often ineffective) skin creams and lotions. Many commercial lotions contain unwanted chemicals and unsaturated oils. Water-based lotions are so readily absorbed by your skin, they leave the skin feeling as dry as it was before they were applied. Because the coconut is covered by several protective layers (the husk, shell, and testa—see section entitled "Parts of the coconut"), even nonorganic coconut oils are fairly free of chemicals, pesticides, and herbicides.

However, if you cannot obtain organic coconut oil, be sure the product you buy is expeller pressed, not refined, so that it is free of chemical solvents.

Just a little coconut oil can go a long way. One of the best times to rehydrate your skin is right after a bath or shower. Don't dry your skin completely. Leave it slightly damp, and then apply a thin layer of coconut oil on the legs, arms, and any other problem areas. If you apply it to your face, don't forget your lips. After you start using coconut oil on a daily basis, you'll notice how water beads on your skin more than it had previously. This is a result of the coconut oil forming a more permanent protective layer on your skin.

If you have trouble with dry skin on the feet, especially cracks around your heels, massage coconut oil into your clean feet before bedtime, then cover them with a pair of clean socks. You'll notice the difference in just a few nights. You also can repair damaged, dry hands the same way using coconut oil and an old pair of white cotton gloves. Finally, coconut oil is much safer for delicate tissues than petroleum-based products, making it an ideal choice as a natural vaginal lubricant. Organic coconut oil is worth the investment for your skin as it will be free of processing chemicals like solvents.

The addition of your favorite aromatherapy oil is an especially nice enhancement. Lavender, chamomile, and rose oils are soothing; peppermint and rosemary are invigorating. Use about fifteen drops for every cup of coconut oil. The eaxct amount of oil depends on the strength of the fragrance and your preference, so add few drops at a time to the coconut oil and rub it the oil on your skin to test.

For easy application, combine the coconut oil and aromatherapy oil in a clean squeeze bottle, such as the small, travel-size containers sold in pharmacies and supermarkets. Prepare a small amount at a time to ensure that the oil essences remain fresh. During the colder months, place your bottle of coconut oil under running hot water if it becomes too thick to use. If you like, cut open and empty out capsules of vitamin E to add to your coconut oil, using about a tablespoon per cup of oil. Vitamin E is an excellent antioxidant and skin healer.

Try this simple exfoliating body rub that moisturizes as it removes dead skin cells and rejuvenates your skin:

2/3 cup brown sugar
1/3 cup warm coconut milk
1 tablespoon coconut oil (optional, for drier skin)

Mix the ingredients in a bowl, and allow to cool. Massage into your skin for several minutes before rinsing. For an invigorating foot rub, try adding 1 to 2 teaspoons of peppermint exact.

For a gentle, safe make-up remover, apply coconut oil with a cotton ball or washcloth.

Massage oil

Massaging with coconut oil is a wonderful way to incorporate this healthful oil into your skin while gaining the benefits of relaxation and touch. Seek out a professional massage therapist or a partner or friend whose touch is soothing to you. If you are able to control the setting for your massage, pick a room that is warm and quiet. Soothing instrumental music will add to the relaxing experience. Although professional massage tables are nice, some thick blankets or several towels on an exercise mat on the floor also can provide a comfortable surface without too much give. A tablespoon or two of coconut oil is all you'll need for an effective massage.

Hair care

Coconut oil is frequently an ingredient in shampoos and hair conditioners. You can apply it directly to your hair about thirty to sixty minutes before you shampoo. Use a few tablespoons to one-half cup depending on the thickness and length of your hair. Begin by massaging the oil into your scalp and letting it drip down. Add more oil if necessary so you can stroke it down the length of your hair with both hands. If you have the time, wrap your hair in a towel, or catch any drips by covering your scalp with a plastic shopping bag, tucking it behind your ears and gathering the ends at the nape of your neck. Let your hair soak up the oil for up to an hour before washing it out. In the summer you can wrap up your hair like this before you go out to work in the garden or yard, letting the warmth of the sun help with the absorption of the oil. It's hard to beat the feel of a soothing, cleansing shower after working outdoors and having a coconut oil hair treatment. Take extra precautions against slipping on the shower floor as you rinse out the oil.

Ultimately, coconut oil should be used in your cooking to feed your skin from the inside out. A nutritious diet that includes high quality, unrefined coconut oil can improve the appearance of hair and skin and give new meaning to the term "beauty from within."

6

Coconut Facts & Tips

The coconut palm is the signature emblem of the tropics. It's difficult to imagine one of these majestic trees without being transported to a soft sandy beach with balmy breezes and ocean waves. This image is not undeserved, as most of the world's coconut palms grow in lowland humid tropics near coastal regions. They also are cultivated in certain inland areas, such as central Africa. These graceful trees can grow up to one hundred feet high and live for sixty to eighty years.

In the sixth century A.D., an Egyptian monk named Cosmas made one of the first references to coconuts found in Western literature. At that time, it was known as the "Indian nut" or "nut of India." The word coconut didn't appear until the era of European exploration after Columbus, when Portuguese and Spanish sailors ventured into previously unexplored tropical areas. The three "eyes" of the coconut shell suggested a grinning face, described by the Portuguese and Spanish word *coco* (grin or grimace).

The Philippines, Indonesia, and India are the largest coconut-producing countries in the world. Smaller crops are grown in other areas of Southeast Asia, as well as the Caribbean, Africa, and Central and South America. Almost half of the world's edible coconut is consumed in the United States and Europe, and about 60 to 80 percent of the dried coconut eaten worldwide is used in baked good, candies, and frozen desserts.

Although the focus of this book is coconut oil, and the thought of coconut itself probably brings to mind a favorite sweet treat, the whole coconut is a source for a surprising array of practical products. It's used to make animal feed, soaps, detergents, emulsifiers, resins and esters, toothpaste, cosmetics, rope, matting, brushes, carpets, fabric, charcoal, furniture, mulch, and housing in tropical areas. Neatly split and cleaned shells are even used for containers.

One of the most innovative uses for coconut oil that we're aware of is as an alternative fuel for diesel engines in cars. Other kinds of vegetable oil have been used to fuel diesel engines, but Austrailian mechanic and inventor Tony Deamer is the first to use coconut oil successfully for this purpose. Living in Vanuatu (formerly known as the New Hebrides), Deamer has solved the problems of thickness, water content, and impurities in coconut oil, opening up the potential for utilizing this plentiful natural resource to replace expensive imported fuel.

Parts of the coconut

Number of countries cultivating coconuts – over 80 First recorded history of coconut – around 300B.C. in India Water content of fresh coconut – approx. 47%

If you're interested in the health benefits of coconut oil, you may want to begin eating more fresh coconut and making your own coconut foods at home. You may come across some unfamiliar terms or confusing information related to the different parts of the coconut.

Coconut kernel or "meat" – This is the white pulp on the very inside of the coconut that is either consumed fresh or dried. Fresh coconut is mixed with water to make coconut cream or milk, or it is dried and pressed to extract the coconut oil. In immature or "young" coconuts, the kernel is smooth and gelatinous and can be eaten with a spoon.

Husk – The husk of the coconut is the outermost layer of the nut as it comes off the tree. On fresh coconuts the husk is greenish, somewhat smooth, and can be two to six inches thick. In supermarkets in the U.S., this layer often is removed to make it easier for consumers to open the nut, but its absence may also lead to a greater chance for spoilage from cracks in the nut shell or damage to the "eyes" at the end of the nut.

Shell – The dark, hard, fibrous covering surrounding the white coconut meat is called the shell. This is what you'll often see when you buy coconuts in a supermarket.

Eyes – At one end of the coconut shell, you'll see three round, smooth areas, each about the size of a quarter, called "eyes." All three of these eyes are viable parts of the female coconut fruit before it is fertilized; once fertilized, only one of the eyes develops. In the section on how to open a coconut in section entitled "How to purchase and open a coconut", it is through this soft permeable "eye" that the coconut water is drained before the shell is broken.

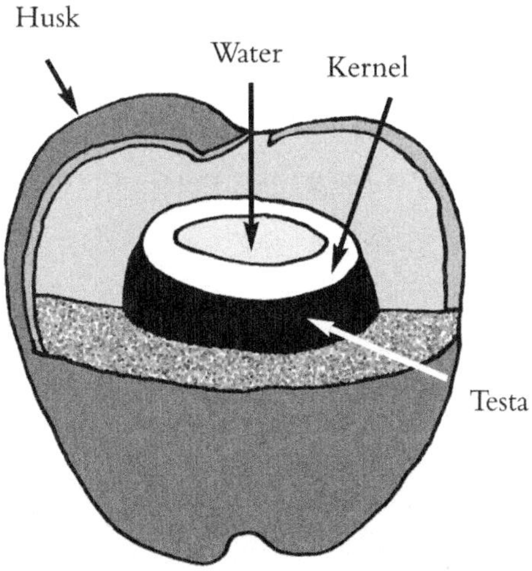

Latin name – *Cocos nucifera*

Average number of coconuts a year from a coconut palm in the wild – 46

Melting point of coconut oil – 24-27°C (75-81°F)

Testa – The thin, brownish skin that attaches the coconut kernel to the shell is called the "testa." This layer often comes off with the coconut kernel when the shell is broken.

Nut – Sometimes the intact, unbroken coconut kernel, removed from the shell with the testa still in place, is simply called the "nut." More often than not, the term is used this way only in reference to commercial processes, but in case you run into it, it refers only to the fresh kernel out of the shell.

Coconut or sap water – People often think that the liquid inside fresh coconuts is what is known as coconut milk, but the term used for this in the commercial coconut industry is "sap water." In cookbooks and other texts for the general public, it is also called coconut water.

Copra – In commercial processes, the coconut kernel is dried to make "copra," then pressed to extract the oil.

Desiccated coconut – This is simply dried coconut, cut and flaked into different sizes.

Coconut milk and coconut cream – As we noted previously, this is not the liquid inside fresh coconuts.

Coconut milk is made by soaking fresh or dried flaked coconut in hot water, then straining out the solids. (See the recipe in section entitled "COCONUT MILK".) Sometimes these coconut solids can be soaked in hot water a second time to make a less rich coconut milk, often called "light" coconut milk. If coconut milk is left to stand, an oil-rich "cream" will rise to the top. When coconut cream is made commercially, fresh coconut kernel often is pressed without the addition of water using special equipment.

On average, one coconut will yield about one cup of coconut cream and one to two cups of coconut milk.

Commercial processes for making coconut oil and other coconut products

The modern commercial method for making coconut oil and other foods from coconut usually involves drying the coconut kernel to make copra. In addition to the coconut kernel, copra also can include some of the parings of the testa and coconut meat that didn't meet the standards for edible coconut. In more traditional processes, this might be done by smoking the crushed coconut kernel, laying it out under the sun, or using large ovens. Because of the mass production involved with either process, the dried copra must be sanitized by bleaching and blanching (a type of pasteurization process). Sometimes it also must be stabilized with sulfites. The oil itself is extracted with solvents (as is done with most commercial vegetable oil processing) and deodorized to make a bland product that will more easily fit the needs of commercial food processors. This type of coconut oil is often called RBD coconut oil (r = refined, b = bleached, d = deodorized).

Omega Nutrition of Vancouver, Canada, and Bellingham, Washington, is an excellent source for organic coconut oil. The company recognized the importance of coconut oil in the early 1990s at a time when it was being "villainized" as a contributor to heart disease. Omega was the first company to reintroduce coconut oil to the health food industry and, combined with the considerable efforts of Dr. Mary Enig, paved the way for many other companies selling coconut oil today. Dr. Enig has worked tirelessly to provide the correct nutritional information on coconut oil and other tropical oils available to consumers.

Omega Nutrition uses a special process to carefully remove the coconut flavor from their oil without using chemical solvents or damaging the oil's healthful properties. The result is a highly versatile product with a neutral flavor that can be used in any recipe. (Many other oils have a distinct coconut flavor which is wonderful in certain dishes but may not be desireable in all recipes.)

Organic oil extraction processes also are springing up in various places around Southeast Asia. Tropical Traditions works with local coconut growers and processors in the Philippines, making a difference not only in the quality of its product but in the quality of life there as well. By using traditional processes that have stood the test of time for centuries to make its coconut oil, the company is able to pass on some of the financial benefits of its operation to small family businesses in the area.

Both Tropical Traditions and Garden of Life, manufacturer of another popular brand of coconut oil, extract the oil by grating the fresh coconut and either pressing the coconut milk from the fresh kernel or lightly drying the kernel and pressing it. Then the coconut milk is fermented for twenty-four to thirty-six hours, at which point the oil rises to the top and separates out from the milk. The oil is then heated slightly to evaporate most of the remaining moisture and filtered to remove any particles that remained from the pressing process. The result is an oil with rich coconut flavor and aroma.

Other organic coconut oil processing operations in Southeast Asia include those set up by the Women in Business Foundation on the island of Samoa, where rural village women also employ traditional methods to make organic coconut oil. In the Caribbean, a brand of oil called Jamaican Gold is manufactured for Essential Oil Company in small batches by cold-pressing organic coconut meat that has been gently dehydrated.

Another commercial process used to make quality coconut oil involves centrifuging the coconut milk made from grated fresh coconut. This separates the oil in the milk from the water and solids and uses no heat. Popular brands using this method are Coconut Oil Supreme and organic Nature's Blessings. There are also other top quality brands of organic coconut oil that are appearing in the marketplace, such as Nutiva, that were manufactured using a variety of processing methods. The growth of this industry attests to the increasing interest in using coconut oil for its health benefits. Please see the list of references for information on how to contact these organizations for their products.

How to purchase and open a coconut

The freshest coconuts are those that have recently ripened on the tree and still have their outer husks intact. Unfortunately, it's rare to find coconuts in this condition in U.S. markets. Without the protective husk, there's more of a chance that cracks can develop in the hard shell or the permeable eye in the shell can be damaged. If that happens, the coconut kernel inside can become rancid. Your best bet is to pick a coconut that still sounds like it has a substantial amount of coconut water inside (shaking a few coconuts will give you some relativity on what this sounds like). Even then, so much time may have elapsed between when the coconut was transported from its original location and it arrived at your market, there's a chance that the inner meat has passed its prime. (An unopened coconut usually will remain good for two to four months.) If you really want to be sure you'll get tasty fresh coconut, you might want to purchase several coconuts at a time to increase your chances that at least one will be excellent.

Before you begin opening your coconut (assuming that you have one with the husk already removed), puncture the permeable eye with an ice pick or screwdriver. A few pokes will easily reveal which of the three eyes is not sealed shut. Wiggle around whatever you insert to widen the hole as large as possible, and invert the coconut over a cup or other container to catch the coconut water inside. Once the coconut has completely drained, you can shatter it open without leaking liquid and creating more of a mess. After you break the coconut apart, rinse any debris from the shattered shell off of the fresh coconut kernel inside.

There are many suggestions for how to open a coconut, and any number of them involves the use of a hammer or cleaver. Many people are successful splitting open a coconut merely by holding it in one hand and tapping it forcefully with a hammer or the side of a heavy cleaver.

If the prospect of hitting a round object with a hard hammer seems daunting to you, a good technique to employ is placing the coconut on the floor wedged into the corner between two walls. Stand with your back to the corner so the force of your blow will drive the coconut toward the corner. If you're concerned about damaging the surface of your corner, pad the side of the coconut against the wall with a thick towel.

My favorite method for opening a coconut was inspired by a number of coconut enthusiasts. Wrap a coconut in a single plastic bag, and insert it in one of those cloth shopping bags available in supermarkets. (I like the added protection the cloth bag gives against shredding plastic.) Two hard whacks against a concrete surface (basement or garage floor, steps, or sidewalk) is usually all it takes to get the job done, and it doesn't require particularly good aim or coordination.

Another method involves baking the drained coconut in either a hot (400°F) oven for fifteen to twenty minutes or a moderate (350°F) oven for about thirty minutes. Sometimes the coconut shell will spontaneously crack with the application of this much heat. Don't heat the coconut for any longer than this or the coconut meat will dry out. Once the coconut has been removed from the oven and cooled, it should split open more easily. The oven method is especially effective for removing the coconut kernel from the shell if it is not separating easily. Alternatively, you can place the pieces shell side down on a cookie sheet, put a little water into each piece to keep the kernel from drying, and bake the pieces in a moderate (350°F) oven for about five minutes. Cool and remove the fresh coconut from the shell.

Once the fresh coconut is out of the shell, the testa or brown rind can be peeled away by hand using a vegetable peeler, although it can be eaten along with the fresh kernel if you don't want to go through this step. Chunks of peeled fresh coconut can be grated by hand using your favorite grater, or it can be processed into smaller pieces or flakes in a blender or food processor. If you can find a coconut grater or shredder, you can leave the coconut meat in the shell and scrape across it to produce flakes or shreds. (See the information in section entitled "SOURCES FOR EDIBLE COCONUT OIL" for how to obtain one of these graters through the mail.)

How to make coconut milk and cream

Coconut milk is a staple of many cuisines in Southeast Asia. With the popularity of Indian and Thai food on the rise in America, more and more people are looking for this ingredient so they can duplicate the delicious flavors they've enjoyed at their favorite restaurants.

To meet this demand, supermarkets are offering a greater diversity of exotic ingredients, so if you live in an urban area, chances are you'll be able to find canned coconut milk. Asian and international markets have long been a source of this product, and you may be able to choose from a wider variety of brands there. Coconut milk also is available by mail through some of the sources in section entitled "SOURCES FOR EDIBLE COCONUT OIL", so if you live in a more rural area, you can stock up.

For freshness, nothing beats making your own coconut milk from scratch. Fortunately this is a relatively easy process.

COCONUT MILK

These are the basic proportions for making coconut milk. You can experiment with the amounts, adding more or less liquid to get the flavor and richness you're looking for. If you use dried coconut, be sure not to use the sweetened, moist coconut often found in bags on supermarket shelves; desiccated coconut is what you'll need.

You'll find a number of recipes in section entitled "Recipes" that call for coconut milk. If you're adventurous, try substituting it for some or all of the liquid called for in gravy recipes, cream soups, milkshakes or smoothies, ice cream, marinades, stews, puddings and cream pie fillings, and the cooking liquid for rice and other grains.

1 cup boiling water, coconut water, or hot milk
1 cup grated fresh or desiccated coconut

Pour the hot water or milk over the coconut in a bowl, and let it steep until it is cool enough to touch. Pour this mixture through a strainer, catching the milky liquid in a bowl or cup and pressing the coconut pulp to extract as much of the rich liquid as possible. Discard the pressed pulp or see the tip for browning it in the Toasting Coconut section on the next page. Refrigerate the extracted coconut milk and use it within two days, or freeze. (The creamy layer that rises to the top can be stirred back in or removed and used in recipes calling for coconut cream; see the section that follows this recipe.)

If the liquid you've extracted is very rich, you might want to try steeping your pulp a second time in another cup of hot liquid, repeating the soaking and draining process as previously described in order to extract a second cup of coconut milk from your batch.

TIP

Both coconut milk and coconut cream make excellent substitutes for dairy products. If you're lactose intolerant or have a dairy allergy, you can make use of these foods in your daily cooking much in the same way you would dairy milk and cream.

If you only want to make a very small batch of coconut milk from fresh coconut, place 1/4 to 1/2 cup of fresh coconut in a blender and add an equal amount of boiling water or hot milk. Process the coconut until it is chopped; then cool it slightly, drain, and press the pulp fairly dry.

To use fewer utensils in the draining process, line a bowl with cheesecloth before adding the grated coconut. Pour over the hot liquid and steep. When the mixture is cool enough to handle, draw up the corners of the cheesecloth, twist the corners around to squeeze the coconut pulp, and press with your hands to extract all the liquid back into the bowl you used for soaking.

COCONUT CREAM

You can find a product in the supermarket or liquor store called "cream of coconut" (used to make piña coladas), but don't confuse this with coconut cream. The two are not interchangeable, as I discovered early on in my experiments with coconut cuisine. Cream of coconut is highly sweetened coconut cream.

There doesn't seem to be an absolute standard for making coconut cream. Traditionally, it is the oil-rich layer that rises to the top of coconut milk. If you refrigerate coconut milk, this creamy layer will solidify at the top of the container of milk, making it easy to remove. In coconut-growing areas, coconut milk and cream also are made by pressing them directly from shredded fresh coconut kernel without adding any additional liquid. You may also hear people refer to "coconut cream" as coconut milk made with dairy milk instead of water, as in the previous recipe for coconut milk.

TOASTED COCONUT

Toasting your own coconut is quick and easy to do, giving you a wonderful condiment for curried dishes or a lightly sweet, nutty topping for desserts. Freshly toasted coconut beats the flavor of the canned product hands down.

To prepare toasted coconut, spread the grated coconut in a thin layer on a cookie sheet and bake it in a 325°F to 350°F oven for five to ten minutes. The only real work is keeping a careful eye on it so it doesn't begin to burn. If you want to make a small amount, a cup or less, this can be done in a toaster oven on a small pan or the broiling tray that came with your appliance.

You also can combine one cup of the coconut pulp left from making coconut milk with several tablespoons of sugar and brown it in a heavy skillet to make a condiment for breakfast and desserts.

NUTRITIONAL PROPERTIES OF COCONUT

per 50g

FRESH COCONUT

approx. 1.6oz., or a 2x2-inch piece, 1/2 inch thick):

calories	177
protein	1.7g

fat	16.8g
saturated fat	14.8g
carbohydrates	7.6g
fiber	4.5g
potassium	178mg
phosphorus	57mg
magnesium	16mg

DRIED COCONUT

3/4 cup

calories	334
protein	3.6g
fat	32.7g
saturated fat	29g
carbohydrates	12g
fiber	17g
potassium	275mg
phosphorus	100mg
magnesium	46mg

7

Recipes

BREAKFAST & BAKED GOODS
SOUPS & SALADS
MAIN DISHES
GRAINS & SIDE DISHES
DESSERTS
DRINKS

COCONUT COOKING MATH

1 coconut = approx. 2 cups grated coconut
1 coconut = 2 cups coconut milk
1lb. coconut = 5 cups grated fresh
1 1/2 tablespoons fresh coconut = 1 tablespoon dried coconut
1 cup grated coconut = 1 1/3 cups flaked coconut = 3 1/2 ounces coconut

Breakfast & Baked Goods

BANANA-COCONUT BREAD

Yield: 1 loaf (16 slices)

Banana bread would surely be on anyone's list of comfort foods. Our version is not only comforting, it's good for you.

1/2 cup coconut oil
1 cup granulated sweetener of your choice
2 cups unbleached white flour
1/2 teaspoon salt
1 teaspoon baking soda
1 1/2 cups mashed bananas (2 to 3 medium)
1/2 cup grated coconut

Preheat the oven to 350°F. Lightly oil and flour a loaf pan, and set aside.

Combine the coconut oil and sweetener in a large mixing bowl. In a separate bowl, mix the flour, salt, and baking soda until thoroughly combined. Alternate adding the dry ingredients and the mashed bananas to the oil and sweetener mixture. Fold in the grated coconut. Pour into the oiled pan and bake for 45 minutes to 1 hour. The loaf will be done when a toothpick inserted in the center comes out clean.

COCONUT COFFEE CAKE

Yield: 9 servings

Bring the goodness of coconut to the breakfast table with this easy recipe. It goes great with a hearty cup of coffee, or my favorite, English breakfast tea.

1/2 cup light brown sugar
2 tablespoons flour
2 teaspoons cinnamon
2 tablespoons coconut oil
2/3 cup grated coconut

3/4 cup sugar
1/4 cup coconut oil
1/2 cup water or coconut milk
1 1/2 cups unbleached white flour
2 teaspoons baking powder
1/2 teaspoon salt

Preheat the oven to 375°F. Lightly oil and flour an 8x8-inch pan, and set aside.

Combine the brown sugar, flour, cinnamon, coconut oil, and grated coconut in a small bowl, and set aside. Combine the sugar, coconut oil, and liquid in a large bowl. Add the flour, baking powder, and salt, and combine well. Spread half of this batter into the prepared pan. Sprinkle with half of the sugar and coconut mixture. Spread over the remaining batter, and top with the remaining coconut mix. Bake for about 30 minutes, or until a toothpick inserted in the center comes out clean. Cool slightly and cut into 9 squares to serve.

BANANA-COCONUT PANCAKES

Yield: 5 to 6 pancakes

These are especially nice in the winter when tropical flavors can brighten chilly mornings.

1 1/4 cups unbleached white flour (can use up to half whole wheat flour)
2 tablespoons granulated sweetener of your choice
2 teaspoons baking powder
1/2 teaspoon salt
1/4 cup grated coconut
1/8 cup coconut oil
1 1/4 cups water or half coconut milk, half water
1 ripe banana, cut into small chunks

Combine the flour, sweetener, baking powder, salt, and grated coconut in a medium mixing bowl. Add the oil and liquid, and combine quickly, leaving some small lumps. Fold in the banana chunks. Heat a griddle or frying pan until a drop of water will bounce over the surface. Lightly oil the pan and ladle on some batter for each pancake, or use a 1/3-cup measure to make smaller pancakes. Bake on one side until bubbles appear on the top of the pancake; flip and bake until browned.

COCONUT-PINEAPPLE WAFFLES

Yield: 4 waffles

Our favorite, tried-and-true waffle recipe can easily be adapted to fit the needs of large or small families. You can cut it in half or double it and still get great results.

1 1/2 cups whole wheat flour
3/4 cup cornmeal
1 tablespoon + 1 teaspoon sugar (optional)
1/4 cup coconut oil
1/2 cup grated coconut
1 tablespoon + 1 teaspoon baking powder
1/8 teaspoon salt
1 1/2 cups pineapple juice

Combine all the ingredients except the pineapple juice in a medium bowl, stirring or whisking well to make sure they are well combined. Add the pineapple juice and set the mixture aside for about 10 minutes, to allow the cornmeal to soften. Ladle into a preheated, lightly oiled waffle iron (vegetable spray does a good job), and bake until firm and lightly browned. Serve with your favorite fruit syrup.

COCONUT FRUIT MUFFINS

Yield: 12 muffins

We think Barb Bloomfield, author of Soups On! *and* Fabulous Beans, *makes the most delicious muffins in the universe—all without eggs and dairy products. Enjoy our adaptation of one of her more memorable creations.*

1 banana, mashed
3/4 cup coconut milk
1/2 cup orange juice
1 1/2 cups whole wheat flour
1 cup unbleached white flour
3/4 cup granulated sweetener of your choice
1 teaspoon baking powder
1 teaspoon baking soda
1/4 teaspoon salt
1/2 cup chopped dates
1/2 cup grated coconut

Preheat the oven to 350°F. Combine the mashed banana, coconut milk, and orange juice in a medium bowl.

Combine the flours, sweetener, baking powder, baking soda, and salt in a separate medium bowl until well mixed. Add to the wet ingredients, stirring just enough to remove any lumps of flour. Stir in the dates and coconut until evenly distributed throughout the mix.

Spoon the mixture into lightly oiled muffin tins, and bake for 15 to 20 minutes, or until a toothpick inserted in the middle of a muffin in the center of the baking pan comes out clean.

Soups & Salads

YELLOW SPLIT PEA-COCONUT SOUP

Yield: 4 servings

Dishes in southern India frequently include the use of coconut. You can enjoy this soup recipe on its own or serve it as a South Indian "sambar" or "kootu" over rice.

1 cup yellow split peas
4 cups water
1/4 cup coconut oil
1 teaspoon turmeric
1/2 teaspoon ground ginger
1/2 teaspoon cumin seeds
1 medium onion, chopped
1 tablespoon chopped fresh garlic
1/2 cup grated coconut

Simmer the split peas in the water until soft and breaking apart, about 45 minutes. Heat the coconut oil in a separate medium sauté pan, and add the turmeric, ginger, and cumin seeds, stirring until the seeds just begin to pop. Turn the heat down to low and sauté the chopped onion and garlic until lightly brown. Toss in the grated coconut and combine. Add the sautéed mixture to the split peas, bring to a simmer, and serve.

COCONUT FRUIT SALAD

Yield: 6 to 7 cups

1 fresh pineapple, cut into chunks (about 4 cups)
2 kiwis, peeled, halved, and sliced
Two 11-ounce cans mandarin orange sections
1/3 cup shredded unsweetened coconut (the larger flakes are great for this)

1 tablespoon fresh lemon juice
1 cup orange juice

Combine the fruit and coconut in a large bowl. Stir the lemon juice into the orange juice, and pour this mixture over the fruit. Cover and refrigerate until chilled.

Main Dishes

NUTTED ANGEL HAIR PASTA WITH GARLIC SAUCE

Yield: 4 servings

My first taste of the original version of this unusual Italian recipe came from a restaurant in Provincetown on Cape Cod. Enjoy this fusion blend of exotic Italian and Pacific flavors.

4 cloves garlic, finely chopped
1/4 cup coconut oil
1/4 cup pine nuts
1/4 cup currants or raisins
2 tablespoons large coconut flakes
1/2 cup Parmesan cheese or nondairy Parmesan substitute

1 pound angel hair pasta

Sauté the garlic in the coconut oil until just lightly browned. Add the pine nuts, currants or raisins, and coconut flakes, and stir to combine. Remove from the heat.

Prepare the pasta until al dente. Toss with the garlic, currants, nuts, and Parmesan, and divide onto four dinner plates.

TOFU VEGETABLE CURRY

Yield: 4 servings

This recipe showcases the Indian practice of tempering spices in oil.

2 tablespoons coconut oil
1 teaspoon cumin seeds
1 teaspoon turmeric
1 teaspoon coriander powder
1/2 teaspoon salt

2 medium carrots, sliced
1 cup frozen peas
1 pound tofu, cut into 1/2-inch cubes
1/4 cup water or vegetable broth
1/2 teaspoon red pepper flakes (optional)
1 cup coconut milk
Salt to taste

Heat the coconut oil in a large, heavy skillet over medium heat. Add the cumin seeds and fry until the seeds just begin to pop. Add the turmeric, coriander, and salt, and sauté for 1 minute. Add the carrots, peas, and tofu, and combine with the spices, cooking for about 5 minutes. Add the water or broth, pepper flakes if using, coconut milk, and salt. Cover and cook over low heat until the vegetables are tender. Serve over brown rice.

THAI FRIED TEMPEH

Yield: 4 servings

If you've never eaten tempeh before, you're in for a taste treat. It's a soy specialty of Indonesia that's especially delicious deep fried. You can find it in the frozen foods section of many natural foods stores.

Two 8-ounce packages tempeh, defrosted if frozen
1 cup coconut oil
1 medium onion, finely chopped
2 cloves garlic, finely chopped
1 teaspoon chili flakes
2 tablespoons minced fresh gingerroot
1/2 teaspoon cumin
1 tablespoon tamari
One 15-ounce can coconut milk

Cut each package of tempeh into four pieces. Using a steamer basket or wire basket, steam the pieces over boiling water for 15 minutes. Remove the tempeh from the steamer, and set aside.

In a medium saucepan, prepare the sauce by sautéing the onion and garlic in 1 tablespoon of the coconut oil until lightly brown. Add the chili flakes, fresh gingerroot, and cumin, and sauté for 2 more minutes. Add the tamari and coconut milk, and heat until just before it boils. Cover and set aside.

Heat the remaining coconut oil in the bottom of a wok. Test the temperature of the oil by dipping in a corner of a piece of tempeh until the oil starts to bubble vigorously. Add just enough of the tempeh so that each piece will float in the oil; it's fine to do only two or three pieces at a time. Turn down the heat if the tempeh begins to brown very quickly. As soon as the pieces are golden, remove with a slotted spoon to drain on paper towels or a wire rack. Continue until all the tempeh has been deep fried. Serve the tempeh pieces over brown rice, and ladle the sauce over.

PACIFIC STIR-FRY OVER RICE NOODLES

Yield: 2 servings

Rice noodles are a wonderful alternative to wheat pasta and are especially good for someone with a gluten allergy. They are not simmered like Italian pasta, but are soaked in hot water instead. Because most of the rice noodles found in the U.S. are imported, there is wide variety in the package sizes and instructions for use, so feel free to adapt the directions given below to fit the product you have on hand.

1 teaspoon sesame oil
2 tablespoons coconut oil
1 medium onion, sliced in half, then in rings
4 cloves garlic, crushed
1/2 pound firm tofu, cut into 1/2-inch cubes
1 green bell pepper, cut into thin strips
1 red bell pepper, cut into thin strips
2 cups sliced Chinese cabbage (approximately 1/2 pound)
1/2 cup shredded coconut
2 tablespoons soy sauce

4 ounces rice noodles

Heat the oils in a wok over medium-high heat, and add the onion rings and crushed garlic. Sauté until just lightly brown. Add the tofu cubes and also sauté until just beginning to brown. Add the bell pepper strips, stirring continuously, and sauté for 5 minutes. Add the Chinese cabbage and sauté another 5 minutes. Stir in the coconut and sprinkle over the soy sauce, combining well. Remove from the heat.

Soak the rice noodles in very hot water according to the package directions (usually for just a few minutes). They will soften quickly. Divide between two dinner plates, and top with the stir-fry.

Grains & Side Dishes

QUINOA AND VEGETABLES

Yield: 4 servings

Quinoa is an ancient grain of South America, high in protein, with a slightly nutty flavor. It has made a comeback into the American food scene over the last twenty years; you'll find it in natural food stores.

1 cup quinoa
1/4 cup coconut oil
2 cups hot vegetarian chicken-style broth
1 green bell pepper, chopped
1 cup broccoli flowerets
1 cup sliced mushrooms

Rinse the quinoa under hot water to remove any natural bitter oils that may be on the surface. Drain well. Heat a large, heavy skillet, and lightly toast the quinoa, stirring continuously, to remove any moisture around the grains. Add the coconut oil to the pan, and sauté the quinoa until just starting to turn golden. Turn off the heat and slowly add the hot broth; do this carefully as the hot quinoa will have the tendency to sputter. Add the bell pepper, broccoli, and mushrooms, and return the pan to low heat. Simmer for 20 minutes, or until all the moisture as been absorbed.

PACIFIC RIM RICE

Yield: 4 servings

A wonderful tropical pilaf.

1 onion, finely chopped
1 green bell pepper, finely chopped
3 tablespoons coconut oil
3/4 teaspoon curry powder
3 cups hot vegetable stock
3/4 cup coconut milk
1 1/2 cups brown basmati rice
1/4 teaspoon salt
1 cup pineapple chunks
1/4 cup chopped cashews

In a 3-quart saucepan, sauté the onion and bell pepper in the coconut oil over medium heat until the onion is golden brown. Stir in the curry powder for 1 minute, then remove from the heat. Slowly add the hot vegetable stock, and bring to a simmer over high heat. Add the coconut milk, rice, and salt. Lower the heat, cover, and return to a simmer. Cook until there is no more liquid visible at the bottom of the pan when you tilt it, about 30 minutes. Remove from the heat, stir in the pineapple and cashews, and let sit for 10 minutes, allowing all the remaining moisture to be absorbed.

ST. LUCIA PILAF

Yield: 3 to 4 servings

The perfect accompaniment to black beans.

1 tablespoon chopped garlic
1 onion, chopped
1/2 cup thinly sliced bell pepper
2 tablespoons coconut oil
2 cups hot vegetable stock
1 cup white basmati rice
1/3 cup currants
1/4 teaspoon salt
1/4 cup chopped Brazil nuts
1 teaspoon grated lime peel

In a 2-quart saucepan, sauté the garlic, onion, and pepper in the coconut oil until the onion is golden brown. Remove from the heat. Slowly add the hot vegetable stock, and bring to a simmer over high heat. Add the rice, currants, and salt. Cover, reduce the heat until the liquid is just bubbling, and cook until all the liquid has been absorbed, about 15 minutes. Stir in the nuts and lime peel, and serve.

MASHED SWEET POTATOES WITH COCONUT

Yield: 4 servings

An easy recipe with uncommonly good flavor.

4 medium sweet potatoes
1 medium onion, chopped
2 tablespoons coconut oil
1/2 cup orange juice
1/4 cup shredded coconut
Salt to taste

Peel the sweet potatoes, cut into quarters, and place in a medium saucepan. Cover with water and simmer until soft. While the sweet potatoes are cooking, sauté the onion in the coconut oil until golden brown. Drain the sweet potatoes and mash. Stir in the sautéed onion, orange juice, coconut, and salt.

COCONUT "BUTTER"

Yield: 1 cup

This spread has a little more flavor than plain coconut oil. It goes well on bread and anywhere else you would use butter.

3/4 cup melted coconut oil

1/4 cup olive oil
2 teaspoons flaxseed oil (optional)

Mix the oils well and keep in the refrigerator.

COCONUT ALFREDO SAUCE

Makes enough sauce for 1/2 pound of pasta

This light alternative to classical Alfredo sauce makes a great accompaniment to fettucine, rice noodles, or your favorite pasta.

1 to 1 1/2 tablespoons fresh minced garlic
2 teaspoons rosemary
3/4 to 1 teaspoon black pepper (amount depends on your taste)
2 tablespoons coconut oil
One 14- to 15-ounce can coconut milk
3 teaspoons cornstarch
2 tablespoons lemon juice
2 teaspoons salt
1 teaspoon onion powder (optional)

In a medium saucepan, sauté the garlic, rosemary, and pepper in the coconut oil until the garlic starts to turn light brown.

Mix the coconut milk and cornstarch separately in a small bowl. When the cornstarch is well mixed, add the coconut mixture to the saucepan, and cook on medium-low heat, whisking frequently. When the sauce starts to simmer, add the lemon juice, salt, and onion powder, if using. Cook until the sauce is thick enough to thickly coat a spoon. Pour over pasta and serve.

Desserts

PUMPKIN COCONUT CREAM PIE

Yield: One 8- or 9-inch pie

This recipe makes use of two Asian ingredients not usually a part of the traditional holiday pumpkin pie: tofu and coconut. Tofu provides the same richness as eggs and dairy products, and coconut adds a nutty undertone that seems just right.

One 12. 3-ounce package firm silken tofu
2 cups (16-ounce can) cooked pumpkin
1/2 cup coconut milk
3/4 cup brown sugar
1 teaspoon ground cinnamon
1/2 teaspoon ground ginger
1/2 teaspoon ground nutmeg
1/2 teaspoon salt

1 unbaked pie shell

Preheat the oven to 350°F. Mash the tofu in the bottom of a large mixing bowl. Add the remaining ingredients and combine with a wire whisk or egg beater. Blend in two batches in a blender or food processor, and pour into a prepared unbaked pie shell.

Bake for about 1 hour, or until the center is fairly firm to the touch. The top may crack just a little. Cool completely on a wire rack, and refrigerate until ready to serve.

THE ULTIMATE COCONUT CREAM PIE

Yield: One 8- or 9-inch pie

Here's a way to make a pie almost entirely out of coconut products! Have a prebaked pie crust ready; the Coconut Flake Crust on the next page or a graham cracker crust are good choices. This pie can take up to six hours to set, so make it early in the day if you plan to serve it that night.

2/3 cup sugar (or equivalent preferred granulated sweetener)
1/2 cup all-purpose flour
1/2 teaspoon salt
One 14- or 15-ounce can coconut milk
1 tablespoon powdered vegetarian gelatin[2]
2 tablespoons coconut oil
1 teaspoon vanilla
1 cup grated coconut

Mix the sugar, flour, and salt in the top of a double boiler before you set it on the stove. Add the coconut milk and cook the mixture in the double boiler, stirring frequently, until it begins to thicken. Stir in the

---

2 Emes Plain Gel is a great product for this. It is vegan and kosher; order from The Mail Order Catalog, listed in the sources section.

powdered gelatin, and remove from the heat. Add the coconut oil, vanilla, and grated coconut.

Let the filling cool slightly, then pour into a prebaked crust. Allow the filling to firm in the refrigerator. (Depending on the type of gelatin you use, it can take from three to six hours.) Top with Coconut Milk "Meringue,", or your favorite whipped topping. (Do not bake this filling with an egg-based meringue; it will liquify if heated.) Sprinkle some toasted grated coconut over the top.

COCONUT FLAKE CRUST

Yield: One 8 or 9-inch pie crust

This is similar to a graham cracker crust, but it uses coconut to replace a large amount of the graham cracker crumbs.

1 cup graham cracker crumbs (approximately 12 crackers) or other cookie crumbs
2 cups coconut flakes
3 tablespoons coconut oil
1/4 cup sugar

Preheat the oven to 350º. Process the graham cracker crumbs and coconut flakes in a blender or food processor until well crumbled. Combine the crumb mixture, coconut oil, and sugar in a bowl until well blended.

Use your fingers to pat the mixture into a pie pan, making sure that it is evenly distributed. Bake for 5 to 10 minutes, until the edges of the crust are brown. Cool completely before adding pie filling.

COCONUT MILK "MERINGUE"

Yield: approx. 2 cups, enough to cover one pie

This is a very simple egg-free meringue. It can take several hours to set (depending on your choice of gelatin), so plan ahead, perhaps making it the night before you want to serve it. This meringue is not baked. It will wilt if warm, so keep chilled.

One 14- to 15-ounce can coconut milk
1/4 cup sugar (or other granulated sweetener)
1 tablespoon powdered vegetarian gelatin[3]

Bring the coconut milk to a simmer in a small pan over medium heat. Add the sugar and gelatin. When all ingredients have dissolved, remove the pan from the heat, allow it to cool slightly, and pour the mixture into a heat-resistant container. Refrigerate until firm; this may take from three to six hours.

After the mixture is firm, scoop into a blender and process until smooth. Pour over a chilled pie ("meringue" may reliquify if pie is warm). Chill for at least one more hour to reset the "meringue."

---

3 Emes Plain Gel is a great product for this. It is vegan and kosher; order from The Mail Order Catalog, listed in the sources section.

HOW TO SET UP A DOUBLE BOILER

If you grew up in a household where the use of a double boiler was commonplace, this kitchen tool will need no explanation. Given today's modern conveniences, however, you may not be familiar with how a double boiler works—or how to improvise if you don't have one. Since a double boiler is called for in several of our recipes, we thought we'd share some tips for its use.

A double boiler will allow you to indirectly heat food. It mainly is used to cook or melt foods that burn easily. You can find double boilers at many culinary stores, but you can also set up a simple version from supplies found in your kitchen. You'll need a heatproof bowl (such as metal or Pyrex) large enough to fit on top of a saucepan, so that the steam from the water boiling underneath will heat the bowl. The bowl should fit the top of the pan so that little or no steam escapes. It should not touch the bottom of the pan or sit in the boiling water. Although the bowl should be heatproof, it should also be a good conductor of heat—not too thick, not made of wood, etc.

When you've found equipment that works, add several inches of water to the saucepan. You'll want enough so that the water won't boil away too quickly, but not so much that your bowl rests in the water. To start the water boiling, leave the bowl on top of the saucepan, or use a separate lid if you need to mix ingredients in the bowl first. You can begin over high heat, but reduce the heat to medium-low once the water boils. Be careful to check the water level occasionally; boiling the water away completely can ruin the bottom of your saucepan. The bowl, as well as the saucepan, will be very hot, and the steam from under the bowl is even hotter, so be cautious when removing the bowl from the saucepan. Use good pot holders (oven mitts are even better), and tilt the bowl toward you as you lift it; this way the steam will escape from behind the bowl and not toward your face.

COCONUT CHOCOLATE BARS WITH ALMONDS

Yield: approx. 2 to 4 dozen pieces

These are reminiscent of Almond Joy bars. They would be a truly unique treat for Halloween.

24 ounces semi-sweet chocolate chips
1 1/2 cups cream of coconut
1 teaspoon vanilla
2 cups powdered sugar
10 ounces shredded coconut (4 cups)
1 cup whole almonds (toasted optional)

Oil a 9x13-inch pan, line with wax paper, and set aside. Melt half the chocolate chips in the top of a double boiler over simmering (not boiling) water. Once fully melted, pour the chocolate into the oiled pan, spreading evenly, and allow to cool.

While the chocolate is cooling, combine the cream of coconut and vanilla in a large mixing bowl. Add the powdered sugar one cup at a time, stirring until completely smooth. Add the coconut and mix briefly.

Spoon the coconut mixture over the hardened chocolate, and pat down lightly. Press the almonds individually into the pan in even rows. Place the pan in the refrigerator until the coconut is hard.

Melt the remaining chocolate chips, and spread evenly over the coconut and almonds. When the chocolate on top is hard, loosen the edges by running a butter knife around the inside of the pan. Turn the pan over onto a chopping board, and gently pull off the wax paper. With the almond side up, cut the bars with either one almond apiece (smaller bars) or two almonds apiece (larger bars).

COCONUT SORBET

Yield: 4 cups

This is best made with the use of an ice cream maker, but also works with hand mixing. It goes well with fruit.

Two 14- to15-ounce cans coconut milk
3/4 cup sugar
1 teaspoon vanilla (optional)

In a small saucepan, mix one can of the coconut milk with the sugar, and simmer over medium heat until the sugar has dissolved.

If using an ice cream maker, add the second can of coconut milk to the rest of the mixture, and cool completely. Follow the directions for your ice cream maker.

If hand mixing, add the second can of coconut milk to the rest of the mixture, cool slightly, and place in a freezer-safe container. Leave in the freezer for 1 hour, then remove and mix by hand with a whisk. Whisk every 30 minutes after that until it is frozen enough to serve.

COCONUT OAT MACAROONS

Yield: 4 dozen cookies

A delicious egg-free version of traditional macaroons.

1 cup coconut oil
1 cup brown sugar
1 cup white sugar
1/2 teaspoon vanilla
1 1/4 cups unbleached white flour
1 teaspoon baking soda
1/2 teaspoon salt
3 cups rolled oats
1/2 cup grated coconut

Preheat the oven to 350°F. Combine the oil, sugars, and vanilla in a large mixing bowl. In a medium bowl, mix the flour, baking soda, and salt until well combined; then stir into the oil and sugar mixture. Add the oats and coconut. Drop by spoonfuls on a greased cookie sheet, and bake for 10 to 12 minutes.

MOLASSES COCONUT CHEWIES

Yield: approximately 4 dozen

Molasses cookies have always been a favorite in our house. The addition of coconut oil and grated coconut makes this flavorful cookie even better for you.

1 cup white sugar
1 cup brown sugar
1 cup chilled coconut oil
2 teaspoons vanilla
1/4 cup molasses
4 cups unbleached white flour, or half white, half whole wheat flour
1 teaspoon salt
1 1/2 teaspoons soda (use 2 teaspoons if using half whole wheat flour)
1 cup grated coconut

Preheat the oven to 350°F. Combine the sugars, coconut oil, vanilla, and molasses in a large mixing bowl. Mix the flour, salt, baking soda, and grated coconut in a separate bowl until well combined. Add the dry ingredients to the molasses mixture, and stir until blended.

Drop by spoonfuls onto an ungreased cookie sheet, and bake for 12 to 15 minutes.

COCONUT DATE BARS

Yield: 18 bars

A healthful treat you can feel good about serving.

1 pound pitted dates, chopped
1 1/2 cups grated coconut
1/2 cup coconut oil
1/2 cup water
1/4 cup liquid sweetener of your choice
2 1/2 cups rolled oats
2/3 cup chopped almonds
1 teaspoon vanilla

Lightly oil a 9x9-inch pan. Combine the dates, coconut, oil, water, and sweetener in a medium saucepan, and simmer for 3 to 4 minutes. Pour into a medium mixing bowl, and add the oats, almonds, and vanilla. Spread in the pan and refrigerate for about two hours. To serve, cut into nine squares, then slice the squares in half to make bars. Store in a tightly covered container.

Drinks

HOT COCONUT CHOCOLATE

Yield: 1 serving

This makes a delicious winter drink.

One 14- to 15-ounce can low-fat coconut milk
2 tablespoons cocoa
5 teaspoons sugar or to taste

Mix the coconut milk, cocoa, and sugar in a small pan over medium heat. When well combined and heated, pour into a mug and enjoy.

CHOCOLATE COCONUT MILK SHAKE

Prepare the Hot Coconut Chocolate as above, combining the ingredients in a blender with 3 or 4 ice cubes. Substituting fullfat coconut milk for the low-fat milk will give you a rich consistency.

Try freezing the mix (without blending with ice cubes) in popsicle trays for an especially good summer treat.

COCONUT MILK SMOOTHIES

Yield: 2 servings

Smoothies are easily done free-form, so use whatever fruit you have in your kitchen. Almost all types will work. (Be wary of seeds, though!) Tropical fruits are perfect for combining with coconut in a smoothie, or try some of the combinations below.

1 to 2 cups fruit of your choice*
One 14- to 15-ounce can coconut milk
3 ice cubes (optional)

Process all the ingredients in a blender, and enjoy!

*Good fruit combinations are:

1 part blueberry to 2 parts peach
1 part mango to 1 part strawberry
1 1/2 cups berry blend (you can find these in your grocer's frozen food section)
1 or 2 bananas—with just about anything!

QUICK PIÑA COLADA SMOOTHIE

Yield: 2 servings

1 cup coconut milk
Two 14-ounce cans pineapple chunks in their juice or 1 1/2 cups fresh pineapple
1/3 cup cream of coconut or 3 tablespoons sugar (optional)

Process all the ingredients in a blender, and top with whipped topping if you like.

GLOSSARY

antioxidants—substances that help prevent the degradation of organic compounds and formation of free radicals

cholesterol—a waxy substance created in our bodies from small molecules of acetate that result primarily from the breakdown of fats and sugars, and in some circumstances, protein

coconut cream—a rich liquid that rises to the top of coconut milk

coconut kernel or "meat"—the white pulp on the inside of the coconut, eaten either fresh or dried

coconut milk—a white liquid made by soaking fresh or dried flaked coconut in hot water, then straining out the solids; can be used much like dairy milk

coconut water or sap water—the liquid inside fresh coconuts

copra—dried coconut kernel

cream of coconut—highly sweetened coconut cream

desiccated coconut—dried coconut, cut and flaked into different sizes *double bond*—a sharing of electrons between atoms, where two atoms contribute two electrons each, for a total of four shared electrons

eyes of a coconut—three round, smooth areas at one end of the coconut shell each about the size of a quarter

fatty acid molecule (free fatty acid)—a chain of carbon and hydrogen atoms with an acid (carboxylic) group on the end; the building blocks of fats

free radicals—unstable molecules that scavenge throughout the body for stable molecules they can raid for oxygen atoms

glycolipids—fats combined with carbohydrates

HDL—the form of lipoprotein that removes fat from artery walls and returns it to the liver so it can be eliminated from the body if not needed

husk—the outermost layer of the coconut as it comes off the tree

hydrogenation—the process used to transform liquid oils into artificially solid fats; hydrogen atoms are added to the double bonds of unsaturated carbon chains, creating a straightened chain without any unstable bonds

lipids—the scientific name for fats and oils

lipoproteins—proteins plus fats

LDL—the form of lipoprotein that transports cholesterol to artery walls to repair damage

medium-chain fatty acids—fatty acids with eight to twelve carbons in their chain

long-chain fatty acids—fatty acids with fourteen carbons or more in their chain

monoglycerides—glycerol plus a fatty acid

monounsaturated fat—a form of unsaturated fat where two carbon atoms along the carbon chain of the molecule share two bonds (four electrons) instead of one bond (two electrons)

nut—the intact, unbroken coconut kernel, removed from the shell with the testa still in place

nutraceutical—a dietary supplement or food that protects against or treats chronic diseases while contributing to better nutrition

omega-3 fatty acids—a polyunsaturated fatty acid required in the diet that lowers blood pressure and reduces inflammation

omega-6 fats—a polyunsaturated fatty acid required in the diet that raises blood pressure and increases inflammation *partial hydrogenation*—when only some of the double bonds in a fat's carbon chain are filled with hydrogen atoms

phospholipids—fats combined with phosphate

polyunsaturated fats—liquid fats that have a chain of carbons where at least two of the carbon atoms are sharing two bonds with at least two other carbon atoms in the chain

RBD coconut oil—coconut oil that has been refined, bleached, and deodorized

saturated fatty acid—a fat made up of a row of carbon atoms that not only are linked together in a chain but are sharing the remainder of their necessary bonds with hydrogen atoms

shell—the dark, hard, fibrous covering surrounding the white coconut kernel

short-chain fatty acids—fatty acids made up of six or fewer carbon atoms

single bond—a bond that consists of two shared electrons, each belonging to a parent atom

testa—the thin, dark brown skin that attaches the coconut kernel to the shell.

trans fatty acids—ats that are manufactured from polyunsaturated fats to have properties that more closely resemble saturated fats

triglyceride—three fatty acids connected to a glyceride molecule; the main form of fat found in the body

unsaturated fatty acid—a carbon chain where at least two of the carbon atoms share two bonds in the chain instead of just one bond

REFERENCES

CHAPTER 3

[1] Sundram, K., et al. "Replacement of dietary fat with palm oil: effect on human serum lipids, lipoproteins and apoliproteins," *British Journal of Nutrition* (November 1992): 68(3):677-92.

[2] de Roos, Nicole M. et al. "Consumption of a Solid Fat Rich in Lauric Acid Results in a More Favorable Serum Lipid Profile in Healthy Men and Women than Consumption of a Solid Fat Rich in trans-Fatty Acids," *Journal of Nutrition* (2001): 131:242-245.

[3] Sadeghi, S., et al. "Dietary lipids modify the cytokine response to bacterial lipopolysaccharide in mice," *Immunology.* (March 1999): 96(3):404-10.

[4] Dunder, T., et al. "Diet, serum fatty acids, and atopic diseases in childhood," *Allergy* (2001): 56:425-428.

[5] Nelson, S.E., et al. "Palm olein in infant formula: absorption of fat and minerals by normal infants," *American Journal of Clinical Nutrition* (1996): 64:291-296.

[6] Cohen, L.A. 1988. "Medium Chain triglycerides lack tumor-promoting effects in the

n-methylnitrosourea-induced mammary tumor model," *The Pharmacological Effects of Lipids,* edited by Jon J. Karbara. Vol III. The American Oil Chemists' Society.

[7] Kabara, John. "Nutritional and Health Aspects of Coconut Oil," *Health Oils* from the Tree of Life.

[8] St-Onge, Marie-Pierre, P.J.H. Jones. "Physiological Effects of Medium-Chain Triglycerides: Potential Agents in the Prevention of Obesity," *Journal of Nutrition* (2002): 132:329-332.

[9] Portillo, M.P., , et al. "Energy restriction with high-fat diet enriched with coconut oil gives higher UCP1 and lower white fat in rats," *International Journal of Obesity and Related Metabolic Disorders* (1998): 22:974-9.

[10] Kaunitz, Hanz, C.S. Dayrit. "Coconut oil consumption and coronary heart disease," *Philippine Journal of Internal Medicine* (1992): 30:165-171.

[11] Kumar, P.D. "The role of coconut and coconut oil in coronary heart disease in Kerala, South India,"

[12] Ng, T.K.W., et al. "Nonhypercholesterolemic effects of a palm-oil diet in Malaysian volunteers," *American Journal of Clinical Nutrition* (1991): 53:1015S-1020S.

[13] Sundaram, K., et al. "Dietary palmitic acid results in lower serum cholesterol than does a lauric myristic combination in normolipemic humans," *American Journal of Clinical Nutrition* (1994): 59:371-377.

[14] Thampan, P.K. *Facts and Fallacies about Coconut Oil,* Jakarta: Asian and Pacific Coconut Community, 1998.

[15] Mendis, S., et al. "The effects of replacing coconut oil with corn oil on human serum lipid profiles and platelet derived factors active in atherogenesis," *Nutrition Reports International* (October 1989): 40:No.4.

[16] Prior, I.A., et al. "Cholesterol, coconuts, and diet on Polynesian atolls: a natural experiment: the Pukapuka and Tokelau Island studies," *American Journal of Clinical Nutrition* (1981): 34:1552-1561.

[17] See note 14 above.

[18] Sadicot, S.M. "Beneficial Effects of Coconut Oil," *Ind. Coco. J.* (1993): XXIV(7):21.

[19] See note 14 above.

CHAPTER 4

[1] Satcher, David. "Emerging Infections: Getting Ahead of the Curve," *Emerging Infectious Diseases* (1995): 1(1):1-6.

[2] Hughes, James M. "Emerging Infectious Diseases: A CDC Perspective," *Emerging Infectious Diseases* (2001): 7(3):494-496.

[3] Mead, Paul S. "Food-Related Illness and Death in the United States," *Emerging Infectious Diseases* (1999): 5(5):607-625.

[4] Bergsson, Gudmundur, et al. "In Vitro Inactivation of Chlamydia trachomatis by Fatty Acids and Monoglycerides," *Antimicrobial Agents and Chemotherapy* (September 1998): 2290-2294.

[5] Petschow, Byron W., et al. "Susceptibility of Helicobacter pylori to Bactericidal Properties of Medium-Chain Monglycerides and Free Fatty Acids," *Antimicrobial Agents and Chemotherapy* (February 1996): 302-306.

[6] Bergsson, Gudmundur, et al. "In Vitro Killing of Candida albicans by Fatty Acids and Monoglycerides," *Antimicrobial Agents and Chemotherapy* (November 2001): 3209-3212.

[7] Wensing, AMJ, et al. "Analysis from more than 1600 newly diagnosed patients with HIV from 17 European countries shows than 10% of the patients carry primary drug resistance:the CATCH study," Report from the 2nd International AIDS Society conference on pathogenesis and treatment, Paris, July, 2003.

[8] Knox, K. Kehl, and Donald R. Carrigan. "Active HHV-6 infection in the lymph nodes of HIV-infected patients: in vitro evidence that HHV-6 can break HIV latency," *Journal of Acquired Immune Deficiency Syndromes and Human Retrovirology* (1996) 11(4):370-8.

[9, 10] Dayrit, Conrad. "Coconut Oil in Health and Disease: ITS and Monolaurin's Potential as Cure for HIV/AIDS." Paper presented at the XXXVII Cocotech Meeting, Chennai, India, July 25, 2000.

BIBLIOGRAPHY

Davis, Brenda, and Vesanto Melina. *Becoming Vegan.* Summertown, Tenn.: Book Publishing Co., 2000.

Dinsdale, Margaret. *Skin Deep.* Buffalo, N.Y.: Firefly Books, 1998.

Enig, Mary. *Know Your Fats.* Silver Spring, Md.: Bethesda Press, 2000.

Erasmus, Udo. *Fats and Oils.* Vancouver: Alive Books, 1986.

Fife, Bruce. *The Healing Miracles of Coconut Oil.* Colorado Springs: Healthwise Publications, 2000.

Fortin, François, ed. *The Visual Food Encyclopedia.* New York: Macmillan, 1996.

Garrison, Robert, Jr., and Elizabeth Somer. *The Nutrition Desk Reference.* New Canaan, Conn.: Keats, 1995.

Gursche, Siegfried. *Good Fats and Oils.* Vancouver: Alive Books, 2000.

Lambert-Lagacé, Louise, and Michelle Laflamme. *Good Fat, Bad Fat.* Toronto: Stoddart Publishing, 1995.

Lombard, Kevin. *Reviewing the Coconut (Cocos nucifera L.).* A paper written and presented for PSS 5326 Advanced Seed Science, Texas Tech University, 2001.

Regional Energy Resources Information Center (RERIC). *Desiccated Coconut Sector.* Klong Luang, Thailand: Asian Institute of Technology, 2002.

Soyatech, Inc. *2004 Soya & Oilseed Bluebook.* Bar Harbor, Maine:Soyatech, Inc., 2003.

Woodroof, J.G. *Coconuts: Production, Processing, Products. 2nd ed.* Westport, Conn.: AVI Publishing Company, Inc., 1979.

SOURCES FOR EDIBLE COCONUT OIL

Essential Oil Company
(Jamaican Gold)
8225 SE 7th Ave.
Portland, OR 97202
800-729-5912
www.essentialoil.com

Garden of Life
770 Northpoint Parkway, Ste 100
West Palm Beach, FL 33407
www.gardenoflifeusa.com

Mid-America Marketing, Inc.
(Coconut Oil Supreme)
P.O. Box 295
Eaton, OH 45320
800-922-1744
www.CoconutOil-Online.com

Alpha Health Products Ltd.
7434 Fraser Park Drive
Burnaby, BC, Canada V5J 5B9
(604) 436 0545
contacts@alphahealth.ca

Nutiva
P.O. Box 1716
Sebastopol, CA 95473
www.nutiva.com

Omega Nutrition
6515 Aldrich Rd.
Bellingham, WA 98226
800-661-3529
info@omeganutrition.com

Tropical Traditions, Inc.
P.O. Box 333
Springville, CA 93265
info@tropicaltraditions.com

Women in Business Foundation
P.O. Box 720, Apia, Samoa
adi@samoa.ws

Nature's Blessings
877-867-4743
orders@naturodoc.com

The Mail Order Catalog for Healthy Eating
P.O. Box 180, Summertown, TN 38483
www.healthy-eating.com 800-695-2241
Organic coconut oil, organic dried coconut, coconut oil skin care products

GRATERS FOR FRESH COCONUT

Tropical Traditions (see above)

Buck's Fifth Avenue
209 5th Avenue SE

Olympia, WA 98501
360-352-9301

BOOK PUBLISHING COMPANY

since 1974—books that educate, inspire, and empower

To find your favorite vegetarian products online, visit:
www.healthy-eating.com

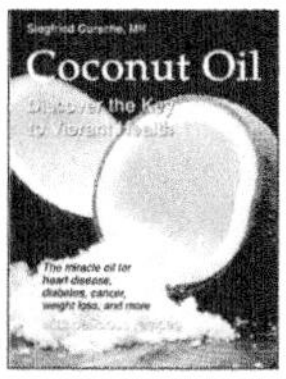

Coconut Oil
Siegfried Gursche, MH

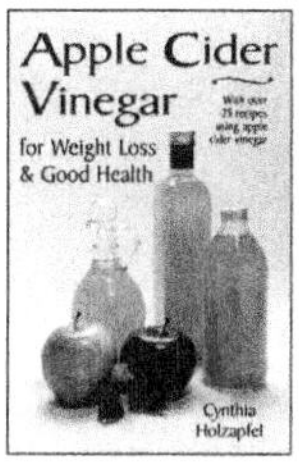

Apple Cider Vinegar for Weight Loss & Good Health
Cynthia Holzapfel

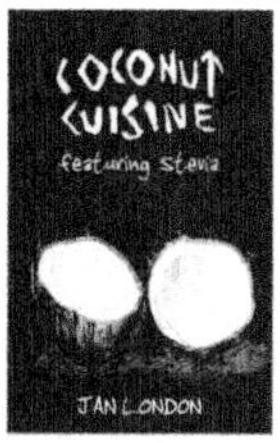

Coconut Cuisine
Jan London

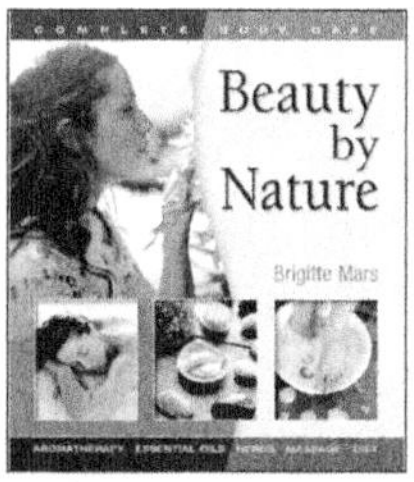

Beauty by Nature
Brigitte Mars

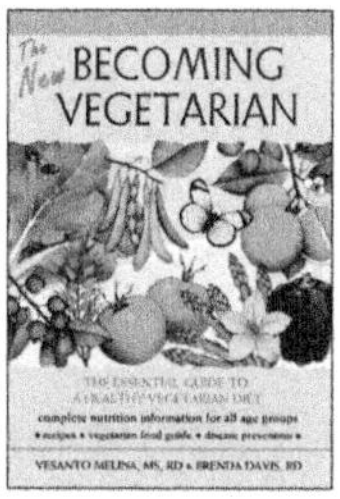

The New Becoming Vegetarian
Vesanto Melina, MS, RD,
Brenda Davis, RD,

Purchase these health titles and cookbooks from your local bookstore or natural food store, or you can buy them directly from:

Book Publishing Company • P.O. Box 99 • Summertown, TN 38483 1-800-695-2241

Back Cover Material

Discover the amazing benefits of Coconut Oil

- Can actually prevent heart disease—does not raise cholesterol levels
- Helps reduce inflammation and immune responses caused by allergies
- Can boost metabolism and help with weight loss
- Easily digested by anyone with ulcers and other stomach and intestinal problems
- Helps to heal wounds and reduce acne
- Kills certain bacteria, viruses, funguses, yeast, and other disease-causing germs
- Has the potential to be an effective tool for fighting HIV infection
- Promotes beautiful skin by protecting against the free radical damage that causes aging

Coconut oil is a stable vegetable oil good for cooking and baking at high temperatures. It can replace hydrogenated vegetable oils that contain harmful trans fats.

Enjoy the light, creamy flavor of coconut oil, along with grated coconut and coconut milk, in recipes for more than 30 flavorful dishes.

A

acne, *58*
adipose tissue, *38*
AIDS, *63, 66, 67, 69*
  therapeutic dose of coconut oil for, *67*
albumin, *22*
Alfredo Sauce, *118*
allergies caused by polyunsaturated fats, *34*
almonds,
  Coconut Chocolate Bars, *127*
alpha-linolenic acid, *8*
American Medical Association, *53*
Angel Hair Pasta, *105*
antibiotics, *50, 51, 53, 54*
  resistance, *50, 51, 53*
  side effects of, *51*
  use in meat industry, *53, 54*
antioxidants, *44*
arachidic acid, *8*
arachidonic acid, *8*
aromatherapy oils, *73*
arterial disease, *44*
avoparcin, *54*
azaserine, *56*

B

bacterial ability to share information, *51*
Banana-Coconut Bread, *95*
Banana-Coconut Pancakes, *98*
benzpryine, *56*
blood sugar levels, *45, 47*
'Butter' Coconut, *116*
butyric acid, *8*

C

cancer, *44, 56*
Candida albicans, *63*
capric acid, *8, 47, 59, 63*
caproic acid, *8*
caprylic acid, *8, 47*
carbon chains, *3, 6*
carotenoids, *20*
Center for Science in the Public Interest (CSPI), *40*
Centers for Disease Control and Prevention (CDC), *51, 53*

chemistry,
  carbon chains, *3, 6*
  electron bonding, *2, 3, 6*
Chlamydia, *59, 61*
Chocolate Coconut Milk Shake, *133*
cholesterol, *20, 21, 22, 45, 47, 66*
  function in the body, *26*
  levels and coconut oil consumption, *41*
  saturated fat and, *29, 30*
Cleveland Clinic, *30*
coconut,
  Alfredo Sauce, *118*
  'Butter', *116*
  Chewies, Molasses, *131*
  Chocolate Bars, *127*
  Coffee Cake, *96*
  commercial processing of, *82, 83, 84*
  consumption per year, *41*
  Cream Pie, *121*
  cultivation and uses, *77*
  Date Bars, *132*
  desiccated, *80*
  eyes, *78, 80*
  Fruit Muffins, *100*
  Fruit Salad, *104*
  how to open, *84, 86*
  how to toast, *90, 91*
  kernel, *78*
  'meat', *78*
  milk, *80*
  nutritional properties of, *91*
  origin of name for, *76*
  Pineapple Waffles, *99*
  shell, *78*
  skin exfoliant, *73*
  Sorbet, *129*
  tips for purchasing, *84*
  water, *80*
  water content of, *77*
coconut cream, *80*
  how to make, *90*
coconut flakes,
  Angel Hair Pasta, *105*
  Coconut Flake Crust, *123*
coconut, grated,
  Banana-Coconut Bread, *95*
  Banana-Coconut Pancakes, *98*
  Coconut Coffee Cake, *96*
  Coconut Date Bars, *132*
  Coconut Oat Macaroons, *130*
  Coconut-Pineapple Waffles, *99, 100*
  Molasses Coconut Chewies, *131*
  Pacific Stir-Fry, *110, 111*

Pumpkin Coconut Cream Pie, 121
Split Pea-Coconut Soup, 102, 104
Sweet Potatoes, Mashed, 116
coconut milk,
(recipe), 87, 88, 90
Alfredo Sauce, 118
Banana-Coconut Pancakes, 98
Chocolate Coconut Milk Shake, 133
Coconut Coffee Cake, 96
Coconut Cream Pie, 121
Coconut Sorbet, 129
Coconut-Pineapple Waffles, 100
Hot Coconut Chocolate, 133
'Meringue', 124
Pacific Rim Rice, 114
Pumpkin Coconut Cream Pie, 119
Smoothies, 134
Thai Fried Tempeh, 108
Tofu Vegetable Curry, 107
coconut oil,
antimicrobial properties of, 57, 58, 59, 61
calories in, 36, 37
as a digestive aid, 34, 36
effect on fatty tissue, 38
effect on metabolism, 37, 38
fatty acids in, 47
for hair care, 73, 75
health concerns over consumption of, 40, 41, 42
in infant formula, 34
to reduce inflammation, 33, 34
for skin care, 71, 73
unfavorable views on,
use in wound healing, 56
coconut oil as a treatment for acne, 58
AIDS and HIV, 63, 66, 67, 69
prostatitis, 36
ulcers, 61, 63
yeast infections, 63
Coffee Cake, Coconut, 96
colitis, 36
cookies and bars,
Coconut Chocolate Bars, 127
Coconut Date Bars, 132
Coconut Oat Macaroons, 130
Molasses Coconut Chewies, 131
copra, 80

corn oil, *41*
Cosmas, *76*
cream of coconut, *90*
  Coconut Chocolate Bars, *127*
  Piña Colada Smoothie, *135*
Crohn's disease, *36*
cryptosporidiosis, *49*
Curry, Tofu Vegetable, *107*

D

Date Bars, Coconut, *132*
Deamer, Tony, *77*
dental carries, *59*
diabetes, *44, 45, 47*
digestion of fats, *20, 21, 22*
docosahexaenoic acid, *8*
double boiler, cooking with a, *125*
double bond, *2*
drinks,
  Chocolate Coconut Milk Shake, *133*
  Coconut Milk Smoothies, *134*
  Hot Coconut Chocolate, *133*
  Quick Piña Colada Smoothie, *135*

E

E. coli, *50, 53*
eicosapentaenoic acid, *8*
electron bonding, *2, 3, 6*
Enig, Mary, *82*
equivalents, for cooking, *94*
erucic acid, *8*
essential fatty acids, *19*
estrogen, *26*
exfoliating body rub, *73*
eyes of a coconut, *78, 80*

F

fats,
  molecular combinations with other substances, *19, 20, 21, 22, 24, 25, 26, 28, 29, 30*
  pathway for metabolism of, *20, 21, 22*
  role in the body, *15, 17*
fatty acid molecule, *8*
fatty acids,
  common food sources of, *8*
  length, *8*
fiber, dietary, *42*
  regulation of blood sugar, *47*
flavonoids, *42, 44*
food borne disease, *49, 51, 53*
free radicals, *28, 44, 70*

Fruit Salad, Coconut, *104*

G

gallstones, *44*
gamma-linoleic acid, *8*
glycerol, *8*
glycolipids, *19, 21*
gram-positive and negative bacteria, *59*

H

hair care, *73, 75*
heart disease, *40, 41, 47*
  role of cholesterol in causing, *28*
  role of saturated fat in causing, *29, 30*
Helicobacter pylori (H. pylori), *61, 63*
high blood pressure, *44*
high-density lipoproteins (HDL), *21, 22, 33, 41*
HIV, *63, 66, 67, 69*
  therapeutic dose of coconut oil for, *67*
hormones, *26*
Hot Coconut Chocolate, *133*
human herpes virus-6A (HHV-6A), *67*
husk, coconut, *78*
hydrogenation, *14, 24, 32, 33*

I

infant formula, *34*
inflammation, *56*
  use of coconut oil to reduce, *33, 34*
Institute of Medicine, *49*

J

Jones, Peter, *37*

K

kidney dysfunction, *44*
Kumar, P.D., *41*

L

lauric acid, *8, 10, 33, 41, 47, 56, 58, 59, 61, 63*
  in mother's milk and baby formula, *34, 36*
linoleic acid, *8, 47*
lipid coated bacteria and viruses, *57, 58*
lipids, *8*
lipoproteins, *19, 21*
long-chain fatty acids, *12, 21, 22, 24*
low-density lipoproteins (LDL), *21, 22, 29, 33, 41, 42*

M

Macaroons, Coconut Oat, *130*

massage oil, *73*
medium-chain fatty acids, *12, 21, 22, 36, 57, 58*
  as an aid in digestion, *34, 36*
  effect on metabolism, *37, 38*
  effect on satiety, *38*
  microorganisms that are destroyed by, *57*
meningitis, *59*
'Meringue' Coconut Milk, *124*
metabolism increased by medium-chain fatty acids, *37, 38*
Milk Shake, Chocolate Coconut, *133*
Molasses Coconut Chewies, *131*
monoglycerides, *20*
monounsaturated fat, *3*
mother's milk, lauric acid in, *34*
Muffins, Coconut Fruit, *100*
myristic acid, *8, 41, 47, 56*

N

nitrosamines, *56*
nutritional properties of coconut, *91*

O

obesity, *45*
oleic acid, *8, 34, 47, 63*
Omega Nutrition, *82, 83*
omega-3 fatty acids, *44*
omega-6 fatty acids, *34, 44, 56*
  and heart disease, *28, 30*

P

Pacific Stir-Fry, *110, 111*
palm kernel oil, *33, 59*
palm oil, *33, 34, 41*
palmitic acid, *8, 33, 34, 47*
palmitoleic acid, *8, 63*
Pancakes, Banana-Coconut, *98*
partial hydrogenation, *14*
Pasta, Angel Hair, *105*
phenolic acids, *42, 44*
phospholipids, *19, 21*
pie,
  Coconut Cream, *121*
  Pumpkin Coconut Cream, *119*
pie crust,
  Coconut Flake Crust, *123*
Pilaf, St. Lucia, *115*
Piña Colada Smoothie, *135*
Pineapple-Coconut Waffles, *99*

plant foods and heart disease, 45
polyunsaturated fat, 6, 34
  health problems with consumption of, 42, 44
Prior, Ian, 42
progesterone, 26
prostaglandins, 19
prostate, enlarged, 36
Pukapuka, 42
Pumpkin Coconut Cream Pie, 119

Q

Quinoa and Vegetables, 112

R

RBD coconut oil, 82
Rice, Pacific Rim, 114
rice, St. Lucia Pilaf, 115

S

Salad, Coconut Fruit, 104
sap water, 80
satiety, effect of medium-chain fatty acids on, 38
saturated fat, 3, 6, 45
  cholesterol levels and, 29, 30
  health concerns about consumption of, 40, 41, 42
Sauce, Coconut Alfredo, 118
saw palmetto, 36
serum cholesterol, 28, 29
sexually transmitted disease, 59
shell, coconut, 78
Shilhavy, Brian, 83
short-chain fatty acids, 12, 21, 22
single bond, 2
skin care, 71, 73
Smoothie, Piña Colada, 135
Smoothies, Coconut Milk, 134
Sorbet, Coconut, 129
Soup, Split Pea-Coconut, 102
Split Pea-Coconut Soup, 102
Sri Lanka, 41, 42
St-Onge, Marie-Pierre, 37
staph infections, 59
stearic acid, 8, 47
Stir-Fry, Pacific, 110, 111
stomach ulcers, 36
Sweet Potatoes with Coconut, 116

T

Tempeh, Thai Fried, 108
testa, 80
testosterone, 26

Thai Fried Tempeh, *108*
Thampan, P.K., *41, 42, 47*
toasted coconut, how to prepare, *90, 91*
Tofu Vegetable Curry, *107*
Tokelau, *42*
toxic shock syndrome, *59*
trans fats, *12, 13, 24, 25, 32*
  assimilation in the body, *25*
  causing high cholesterol levels, *28*
  heart disease and, *33*
triglycerides, *8, 10, 12, 21*
tropical oils, health concerns about consumption of, *40, 41, 42*
Tropical Traditions, *83*
tuberculosis, *53*

U

ulcers, *59*
  coconut oil for treatment of, *61, 63*
uncoupling protein (UCP1), *38*
unsaturated fat, *3, 6, 70, 71*

V

vitamin A, *19, 20*
vitamin D, *20, 26*
vitamin E, *20, 44, 47*
vitamin K, *20*
vitamins, metabolism of, *19, 20*

W

Waffles, Coconut-Pineapple, *99*
weight loss, *36, 37, 38*
Willett,Walter, *29*
Women in Business Foundation, *83*
World Health Organization, *54*

Y

yeast infections, *63*
'young' coconuts, *78*

Printed in Dunstable, United Kingdom

91220086R00098